Dementia

KARGER

Printed in Switzerland
on acid-free paper by
Thür AG Offsetdruck, Pratteln

Appears bimonthly:
1 volume per year (6 issues)

Dementia

Submission: Only original papers written in English are considered and should be sent to:

S. Karger AG
Editorial Office 'Dementia'
P.O. Box
CH-4009 Basel (Switzerland)

papers from USA/Canada to be sent to:

S. Karger Publishers, Inc.
Editorial Office 'Dementia'
26 West Avon Road
P.O. Box 529
Farmington, CT 06085 (USA)

Manuscripts should be submitted in triplicate (with three sets of illustrations of which one is an original), typewritten double-spaced on one side of the paper, with a wide margin.

Conditions: All manuscripts are subject to editorial review. Manuscripts are received with the explicit understanding that they are not under simultaneous consideration by any other publication. Submission of an article for publication implies the transfer of the copyright from the author to the publisher upon acceptance. Accepted papers become the permanent property of 'Dementia' and may not be reproduced by any means, in whole or in part, without the written consent of the publisher. It is the author's responsibility to obtain permission to reproduce illustrations, tables, etc. from other publications. The manuscripts should be accompanied by a statement by the submitting author certifying that all the authors have read the papers and have agreed to having their names listed as authors. A similar statement should be appended for the names of colleagues who are acknowledged in footnotes as having contributed to or criticized the paper. For papers involving human subjects, adequate documentation should be provided to certify that appropriate ethical safeguards and protocols have been followed. Animal experiments should include a clear description of the method of anesthesia and killing.

Arrangement: All pages should be consecutively numbered beginning with the title page, then the text, acknowledgements, references and legends to figures. Two types of manuscripts will be considered:
1. Original Research Articles. An Abstract, Introduction, Materials and Methods, Results, and Discussion sections are required. The literature review should be succinct. There are no restrictions on the number of pages or figures.
2. Review Articles in which a specific field is reviewed through an exhaustive literature survey. An Abstract is required. A Materials and Methods section and a Results section are not required. There are no restrictions on the number of pages or figures. Preliminary notes are not desired.
Title page: The first page of each paper should indicate the title (main title underlined), the authors' names, and the institute where the work was conducted. A short title for use as running head as well as the full address of the author to whom correspondence should be sent are also required.
Full address: The exact postal address complete with postal code must be given at the bottom of the title page. Please also supply phone and fax numbers.
Key words: For indexing purposes, a list of 3–10 key words in English is essential. Try to use key words such as found in the headings of Index Medicus.
Abstract: The first page of the text should include an abstract of up to 10 lines.
Small type: Paragraphs which can or must be set in smaller type (case histories, test methods, etc.) should be indicated with a 'p' (petit) in the margin on the left-hand side.
Footnotes: Avoid footnotes. When essential, they are numbered consecutively and typed at the foot of the appropriate page.
Abbreviations: Abbreviations should not be used excessively in the text. Only standard abbreviations should be used. Nonstandard abbreviations of terms that are used frequently in the text should be explained by the term written out completely and followed immediately by the abbreviation in parentheses, for example: 'increase in norepinephrine (NE) content . . .'.
Tables and illustrations: Tables and illustrations (both numbered in Arabic numerals) should be prepared on separate sheets. Tables require a heading and figures a legend, also prepared on a separate sheet. For the reproduction of illustrations, only good drawings and original photographs can be accepted; negatives or photocopies cannot be used. When possible, group several illustrations on one block for reproduction (max. size 181 × 223 mm) or provide crop marks. On the back of each illustration, indicate its number, the author's name, and 'top'. Color illustrations are reproduced at the author's expense. Illustrations from manuscripts to be contained in an issue will be considered for publication on the front cover.
References: In the text identify references by Arabic numerals [in square brackets]. Material submitted for publication but not yet accepted should be noted as 'unpublished data' and not be included in the reference list. The list of references should include only those publications which are cited in the text. Do not alphabetize; number references in the order in which they are first mentioned in the text. The surnames of the authors followed by initials should be given. There should be no punctuation other than a comma to separate the authors. Cite all authors, 'et al' is not sufficient. Abbreviate journal names according to the Index Medicus system. (Also see International Committee of Medical Journal Editors: Uniform requirements for manuscripts submitted to biomedical journals. Br Med J 1988;296:401–405.)
Examples
(a) Papers published in periodicals: Alzheimer A: Über eine eigenartige Erkrankung der Hirnrinde. Neurol Centralbl 1907;18:177–179.
Goldgaber D, Lerman MI, McBride OW, Saffiotti U, Gajdusek DC: Characterization and chromosomal localization of a cDNA encoding brain amyloid of Alzheimer's disease. Science 1987;235: 877–884.
(b) Monographs: Matthews DE, Farewell VT: Using and Understanding Medical Statistics. Basel, Karger, 1985.
(c) Edited books: Esiri MM: Typical and atypical viruses in the aetiology of senile dementia of the Alzheimer type; in Ulrich J (ed): Histology and Histopathology of the Aging Brain. Interdiscipl Top Gerontol. Basel, Karger, 1988, vol 25, pp 119–139.
Further details: Authors may consult our leaflet 'Rules for the Preparation of Manuscripts', available on request from the Publisher, S. Karger AG, P.O. Box, CH-4009 Basel (Switzerland).

Page charges: There is no page charge for papers of 5 or fewer printed pages (including tables, illustrations and references). Each additional complete or partial page is charged to the author at SFr. 225.–/US $ 150.00. The allotted size of a paper is equal to approx. 15 manuscript pages (including tables, illustrations and references). These charges will commonly be levied but are not a prerequisite to the publication of any article.

Galley proofs: Unless indicated otherwise, galley proofs are sent to the first-named author and should be returned with the least possible delay. Alterations made in galley proofs, other than the correction of printer's errors, are charged to the author. No page proofs are supplied.

Reprints: Order forms and a price list are sent with the galley proofs. Orders submitted after the issue is printed are subject to considerably higher prices. Allow five weeks from date of publication for delivery of reprints.

KARGER

General Information

Dementia

Publication data: 'Dementia' is published 6 times annually. Volume 4 with 6 issues appears in 1993.

Subscription rates: Subscriptions run for a full calendar year. Prices are given per volume.

Personal subscription:

Subscription + postage and handling
SFr. 141.– + SFr. 5.30 Europe
SFr. 141.– + SFr. 8.– Overseas
US$ 94.00 + US$ 5.30
(Must be in the name of, billed to, and paid by an individual. Order must be marked 'personal subscription'.)

Institutional subscription:

Subscription + postage and handling
SFr. 637.– + SFr. 24.– Europe
SFr. 637.– + SFr. 36.– Overseas
US$ 425.00 + US$ 24.00

Airmail postage: SFr. 36.–, US$ 30.00.
(Extra per volume.)

Microform edition: SFr. 318.50, US$ 212.50.
(Available exclusively to subscribers of the paper edition.)

Subscription orders: Orders can be placed at agencies, bookstores, directly with the Publisher S. Karger AG, P.O. Box, CH – 4009 Basel (Switzerland) or with any of the following distributors:

Deutschland: S. Karger GmbH, Postfach
D – 79095 Freiburg

France: Librairie Luginbühl
36, bd de Latour-Maubourg, F–75007 Paris

Great Britain, Ireland: S. Karger Publishers
11 Ravenscroft Road
Beckenham, Kent BR3 4TP

USA: S. Karger Publishers, Inc.
26 West Avon Road, P.O. Box 529
Farmington, CT 06085

India, Bangladesh, Sri Lanka:
S. Karger India Subscription Agency
B – 5/132 Safdarjung Enclave
New Delhi-110029

Japan: Katakura Libri, Inc.
36-9 Hongo 3-chome, Bunkyo-ku, Tokyo 113

Change of address: Both old and new address should be sent to the subscription source.

Single issues and back volumes: Information can be obtained through the Publisher.

Advertising: Correspondence and rate requests should be addressed to the Publisher.

Bibliographic indices: This journal is regularly listed in bibliographic services, including *Current Contents®*.

Book Reviews: Books are accepted for review by special agreement.

Guidelines for Disk Submission

Karger Publishers welcomes the submission of manuscripts on disk.

Please observe the 'Instructions to authors' as well as the following guidelines:

Technical Data

The preferred **storage medium** is a 3.5- or 5.25-inch disk in MS-DOS format. Macintosh is also acceptable.

The preferred **word processing package** is Microsoft Word. Other commonly used PC text programs are also accepted, as well as ASCII formats.

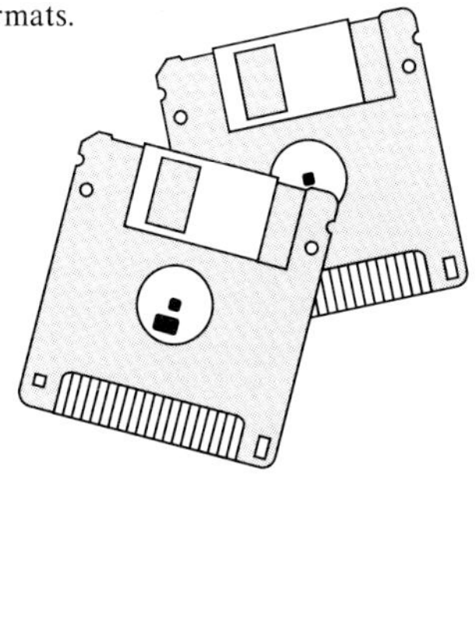

Handling

All manuscripts accepted for Karger publications are subject to copy editing. It is therefore essential that you send us a **double-spaced printout** of your manuscript which exactly matches the disk.

Any subsequent revised versions should be clearly marked as such, both on the disk and on the manuscript.

The copy-edited manuscript and the disk will be returned to you along with the galley proofs. Please be sure to **check the galleys against the manuscript** in which changes introduced by the copy editor and/or questions will be marked.

Please **label** your disk with (a) the title of the journal for which it is submitted, (b) a short version of the paper title, (c) your name and (d) the software and hardware used.

Text Arrangement

Text and headings should be ranged left throughout, without word breaks. **Do not center, space, or use block letters** for text and headings (except for abbreviations).

Do not use indentations to mark the beginning of a paragraph, but use one blank line between paragraphs.

Be sure to use the **same type style for headings of the same ranking** throughout the text.

When using **special characters** not available on a standard keyboard (including Greek characters), please do so by a readily identifiable code, and use the same code throughout the manuscript. Supply a **complete list of the codes used** at the beginning of the text.

Illustrations, tables and mathematical formulae will be handled conventionally.

KARGER

The 2nd International Conference on Frontal Lobe Degeneration of Non-Alzheimer Type

Guest Editor
Arne Brun, Lund, Sweden

September 11–12, 1992
Lund, Sweden

35 figures, 37 tables, 2 colour plates, 1993

KARGER

S. Karger
Medical and Scientific Publishers
Basel · Freiburg · Paris · London
New York · New Delhi · Bangkok
Singapore · Tokyo · Sydney

Drug Dosage
The authors and the publisher have exerted every effort to ensure that drug selection and dosage set forth in this text are in accord with current recommendations and practice at the time of publication. However, in view of ongoing research, changes in government regulations, and the constant flow of information relating to drug therapy and drug reactions, the reader is urged to check the package insert for each drug for any change in indications and dosage and for added warnings and precautions. This is particularly important when the recommended agent is a new and/or infrequently employed drug.

P.O. Box, CH-4009 Basel (Switzerland)
Printed in Switzerland on acid-free paper by
Thür AG Offsetdruck, Pratteln
ISBN 3-8055-5824-4

Contents

Dementia 1993;4:125

Arne Brun

Guest Editor, Lund

Dementia of Frontal Type

During the last 10 years, dementia of frontal lobe type has been recognized as a variant of progressive dementia. A number of disorders affecting the frontal lobes, either primarily or secondarily, are known to cause progressive behavioural dysfunction and eventually produce full dementia.

A congress highlighting this theme, held in Lund, Sweden 1986, defined a form of presenile dementia with primary degenerative involvement of the frontal cortex. A second congress on frontal dementia was held in the same city in 1992. The second conference was arranged by the Dementia Study Group, University of Lund, Sweden in collaboration with the French Foundation for Alzheimer Research (Los Angeles, Calif., USA) and sponsored, in part, also by the Crafoord Foundation (Lund, Sweden), and contributions to this meeting are featured in this issue of *Dementia.*

In the past, frontal dementia has been synonymous with Pick's disease, a progressive degenerative disorder involving the frontal and temporal cortex. To this can be added frontal dementia of non-Alzheimer type (FLD), a relatively common problem, plus a progressive language dysfunction with frontal lobe atrophy with the same pathology as FLD and also a frontal dementing syndrome lacking distinct histopathology. Presenile dementia associated with motor neuron disease represents yet another disorder that can produce frontal cortical pathology. These entities form a group of disorders that are related with respect to the cortical site of structural change. Other disorders with more widespread pathological background can also produce 'frontal' symptomatology; these form a group of secondary frontal dementias. A variety of degenerative vascular, toxic and infectious disorders, all apparently involving subcortical structures with strong frontal connections, can be included in this 'secondary' group. Here the subcortical abnormalities appear to be the source of 'frontal system disorders'.

Among the *primary cortical disorders,* the largest single group are those with FLD. Pathoanatomically, these cases show degeneration of the superficial layers of the frontal and anterior temporal cortex with mild gliosis and microvacuolation, but have neither Pick nor Alzheimer core changes. FLD is markedly familial but, to date, genetic linkage has not demonstrated the site of the abnormal gene. The possibility of a prion abnormality has neither been validated nor disproved in FLD or Picks's disease.

Regional brain isotope studies (SPECT, PET and rCBF) verify the frontal malfunction. One series has suggested greater right hemisphere involvement, an asymmetry noted in both FLD and Pick's disease. The progressive nature of FLD has been shown by serial blood flow measurements performed over several years. The degree of cognitive impairment parallels the reduction in cerebral blood flow in fronto-temporal areas, and both are consistent with the pathological findings. Behavioural activation of FLD patients produced augmentation of flow in the frontal areas but not to the level of normality.

Recognition of frontal degenerative disorders is important for research in other dementing diseases, including Alzheimer's disease, where the frontal dementias may be an important confounding factor. The effects of ageing and of the disorders that accompany ageing demand attention when judging the cognitive impaiments and the blood flow decline in FLD. Hopefully, future investigations will throw light on the nature of the degenerative frontal lobe dementias with respect to their nature and etiology, making a more precise classification possible and paving the way for future treatment.

Prof. Arne Brun, MD, PhD
Department of Pathology
Division of Neuropathology
University Hospital
S-221 85 Lund (Sweden)

1013-7424/93/0044-0125
$2.75/0

Dementia 1993;4:126–131

Arne Brun

Neuropathology Division, Institute of Pathology, University Hospital, Lund, Sweden

Frontal Lobe Degeneration of Non-Alzheimer Type Revisited

Key Words
Neurodegeneration
Frontal lobe degeneration
Non-Alzheimer dementia

Abstract
The neuropathology of frontal lobe degeneration of non-Alzheimer type was reevaluated on the basis of a new material of 13 cases against the background of experiences from earlier published 16 cases. The salient neuropathological feature was an unspecific neuronal degeneration of superficial cortical layers of the frontal and to some extent the temporal lobes without markers for Alzheimer's, Pick's or Lewy body diseases and there were no indications so far of a prion etiology. The consistency of histopathological features are taken to indicate a disease entity, also identified by other authors. It is tentatively grouped together with progressive and aphasic dementia, similar cases in the literature and possibly also Pick's disease and ALS with dementia.

Introduction

Frontal lobe degeneration (FLD) of non-Alzheimer type was in 1987 patho-anatomically defined [1] as a mainly frontal and limited anterior temporal cortical degeneration, grossly with no discernible or only mild atrophy that also involved mainly the anterior portion of the cingulate gyrus. Histologically it was characterized by gliosis, mild neuronal loss and microvacuolation of lamina I–III. There were no Alzheimer changes except mild ones compatible with age, no amyloidosis and no Pick bodies or inflated neurons. The amygdala, hippocampus and striate body were not or only mildly involved and over all there were no changes in the thalamus or globus pallidus. Also the substantia nigra usually showed no or mild changes. In the white matter there was a mild gliosis [2]. FLD was then tentatively launched as an entity which went with a neuropsychiatric picture [3] and regional cerebral blood flow decrement [4] matching the pathology. Since then this disease has been repeatedly observed and the aim of the present study is to further characterize it, and to study its relation to similar conditions described in the literature and met with in our material.

Material and Methods

The new material consists of 13 cases (tables 1, 2) which are compared to 1 case of ALS with dementia, and 2 cases of Pick's disease (table 3). These are contrasted with 27 cases with a frontal symptomatology but with different disorders of differential diagnostic interest (table 4). These 43 cases are all derived from a prospective longitudinal dementia study of 240 cases during the years 1986–1992, the material in its entirety now encompassing 400 cases (fig. 1) [Gustafson, this volume]. They had all been subject to a psychiatric, neuropsychological and regional cerebral blood flow study, accounted for in subsequent papers of this volume [Gustafson, Risberg].

Neuropathologically the brains were extensively studied in whole brain coronal semiserial sections, and stained for microscopy with basic neuropathological methods employed in previous studies, supplemented with prion antibodies (kindly supplied by Dr. S. Prusiner, San Francisco, Calif., USA), ubiquitin for protein degradation products, and parallel methods such as Gallyas and Campbell's methods for neuritic degeneration, plaques, tangles and amyloid. Some of the cases were also analyzed with molecular biological methods regarding the prion gene. The extensive microscopical analysis allowed a safe recording of type of change and its severity and distribution but also the presence or absence of other pathological changes of importance for clinico-pathological correlations.

Arne Brun, MD, PhD
Department of Pathology
Division of Neuropathology
University Hospital
S–221 85 Lund (Sweden)

1013–7424/93/0044–0126
$2.75/0

Table 1. Distribution of changes in FLD of non-Alzheimer type

No.	Sex	Age	Br wt	Fro	Centr	Temp	Par	Occ	Ins	Gy cing ant/post	Am	Hipp	CS	Th	GP	Cere-bell	SN
1	F	76	835	++	–	++	(+)	–	+	+/+	+	–	(+)	–	–	–	(+)
2	F	51	1,440	++	–	–	(+)	–	+	+/–	–	–	(+)	–	–	–	+
3	M	68	–	++	–	++	–	–	NS	NS	NS	NS	NS	NS	NS	NS	NS
4	M	61	1,100	++	(+)	++	+	–	+	+/–	+	(+)	+	–	+	–	+
5	F	56	1,620	++	++	+	–	–	+	+/+	+	+	+	–	–	(+)	++
6	M	69	1,230	+	–	++	(+)	–	+	+/+	++	(+)	(+)	–	–	(+)	–
7	M	74	1,270	+	–	(+)	–	–	(+)	+/–	–	–	–	–	–	+	+
8	F	59	935	++	(+)	(+)	(+)	(+)	+	+/+	(+)	–	(+)	–	–	–	(+)
9	M	60	1,200	++	–	(+)	(+)	–	–	+/–	–	–	–	–	–	–	++
10	M	50	1,030	++	+	–	(+)	–	–	+/–	–	–	–	–	–	–	(+)

Br wt = Brain weight; Fro = frontal cortex; Centr = central, pre- and postcentral gyri; Temp = temporal anterior 1/3; Par = parietal cortex; Occ = occipital cortex; Ins = insula; Gyr cing = cingulate gyrus; Am = amygdalar nucleus; Hipp = hippocampus; CS = corpus striatum; Th = thalamus; GP = globus pallidus; Cerebell = cerebellar cortex; SN = substantia nigra; NS = not studied.

Neuropathological Results

Out of the 43 cases 10 were diagnosed as FLD (table 1), 1 as ALS with FLD, 3 as probable advanced FLD (table 2), 2 as Pick's disease (table 3) and 27 cases had disorders of various types but with frontal accent with a more or less elusive clinical FLD character (table 4).

FLD of Non-Alzheimer Type

The 10 cases with FLD listed in table 1 (F/M = 4/6, age range 51–76) in all but 2 cases showed none to moderate loss of brain weight and grossly a mild to not discernable atrophy of the frontal and temporal lobes without circumscribed or knifeblade type of shrinkage. On cutting the brains showed no striking changes except for a mild widening of the frontal ventricular horns. The cortical degeneration was asymmetric in 4 of the cases. Microscopically there was a degeneration in the cortex limited to the superficial layers. The changes were of a nonspecific type with mild loss of neurons, microvacuolation and astrocytic gliosis (fig. 1, 2). These alterations were most pronounced in the anterior portions of the frontal convexity cortex without prominent involvement of the subfrontal cortex, and subsidizing towards the central gyri, and also seen in the anterior 1/3 of the temporal lobe though less pronounced. It also involved the insula and the cingulate gyrus, in half of the cases only in its anterior portion and in the remaining more pronounced cases also in its posterior half. The central, parietal and occipital areas showed none to very mild changes of the same type. Except in 1 case the amygdala was not or only very mildly

Table 2. Advanced FLD

No.	Sex	Age	Diagnosis
1	F	62	Widespread cortical changes; advanced FLD
2	F	75	Intense cortical degeneration; advanced FLD
3	M	51	Widespread cortical degeneration involving also striatum, hypothalamus, but not hippocampus and amygdala; advanced FLD

Table 3. Pick's disease

No.	Sex	Age	Diagnosis
5	F	62	Pick's disease
6	F	42	Pick's disease

Table 4. Other pathology behind disorders with clinical similarities to FLD (1986 and 1992 materials)

	1992	1986	Total
DAT with frontal accent with or without leukoencephalopathy	9	2	11
Bilateral thalamic infarct		1	1
Jakob-Creutzfeldt's disease	1	3	4
Frontal traumatic encephalopathy	2		2
SIWI, pure	5		5
Binswanger	4		4
Total	21	6	27

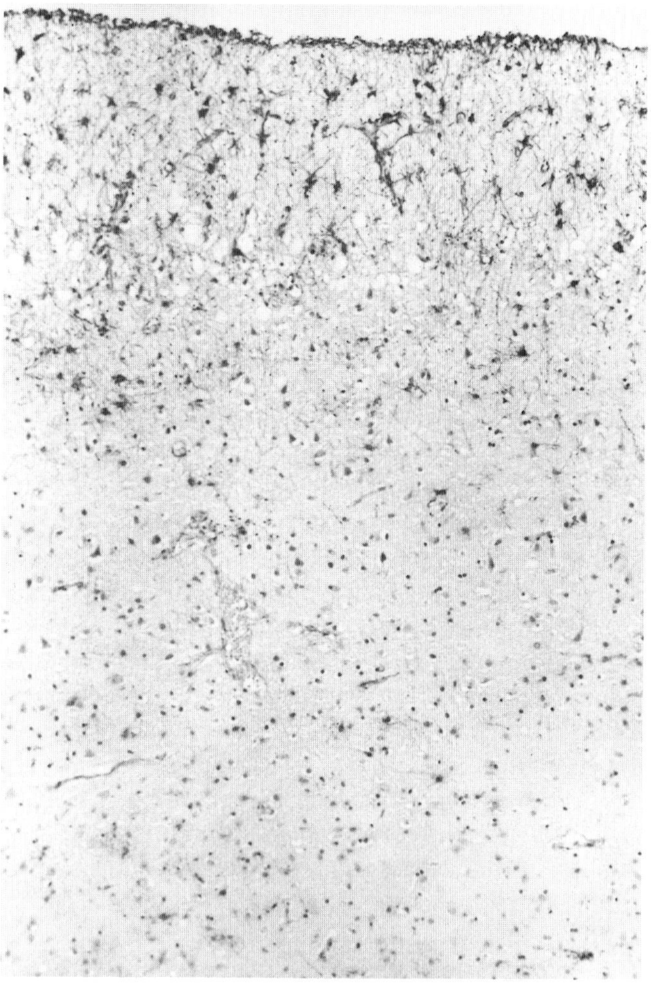

Fig. 1. Frontal cortex, Brodmann area 10, showing cortical layers I–IV. Pathological changes seen only in layers I to superficial layer III with microvacuolation and dense dark astrocytes as revealed by the immunostaining for GFAP. × 80.

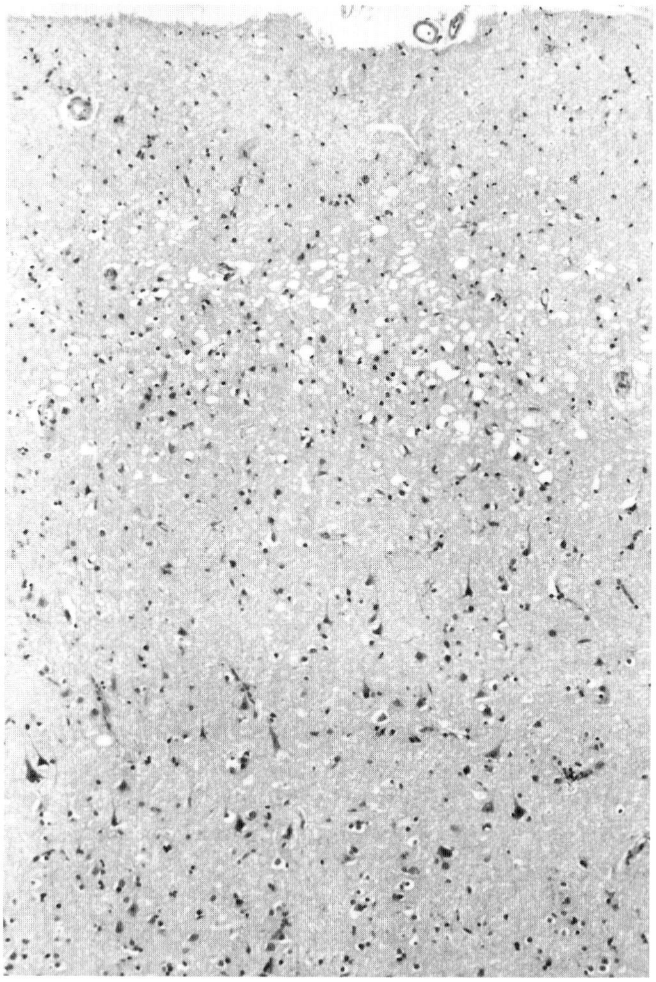

Fig. 2. Frontal cortex, Brodmann area 10, showing layers I–III with neuronal loss and microvacuolation in lamina II and superficial lamina III. Hematoxylin and eosin. × 100.

involved and the hippocampus never showed obvious changes. The striate body was very mildly involved only in 5 of the cases whereas the globus pallidus and thalamus appeared normal. The nucleus basalis Meynert showed mild changes in only 2 of the cases. The cerebellum was largely normal and in the substantia nigra there was a moderate degeneration in 2 cases but mild or insignificant in the others. The cervical cord was unremarkable (table 1).

There were neither plaques nor tangles or amyloid angiopathy except for in the older cases where it was fully compatible with physiological age changes. In a few of the cases there were, however, diffuse amyloid deposits with Campbell's method and antibodies to β-amyloid and sparse occurrence of dystrophic neurites with Gallyas method, also shown with ubiquitin. There were however no Lewy bodies. Antiprion antibodies showed no prion deposits and the cases studied with molecular genetic methods had no abnormal prion gene [5]. Antibodies to gliofibrillar acid protein (GFAP) revealed astrocytic gliosis distinctly limited to layers I to III (fig. 1) in most areas, only in some places extending further down into the cortex. This pattern was repeated with ubiquitin giving a positive reaction in layers I, II and superficial portions of layer III but not in deeper layers. In the white matter there was a very mild loss of myelin in the frontal white matter and a mild astrocytic gliosis, probably secondary to the myelin loss. Blood vessels were unremarkable.

Advanced Probable FLD of Non-Alzheimer Type

In this group there are 3 cases (table 2), who showed changes identical to those found in FLD, only more widespread appearing also in the parietal and occipital cortex, in areas more penetrating towards inferior cortical layers and in case number 3 with more prominent degenerative changes, e.g. in the striatum and substantia nigra. For these reasons they are for the time being kept apart from the group of 10 FD cases (table 1).

ALS with FLD

A 55-year-old lady with amyotrophic lateral sclerosis, with the classical findings in the spinal cord and muscles, showed no gross brain atrophy but on microscopy cortical changes as found in FLD, again without Alzheimer changes or only a very mild amyloid angiopathy, no Pick cells and no Lewy bodies. This case is an example of motor neuron disease with dementia as described in the literature.

Pick's Disease

The 2 cases of Pick's disease (table 3), 2 females aged 62 and 42, respectively, showed the typical circumscribed severe frontal atrophy seen in morbus Pick, severe basal ganglia atrophy, Pick bodies and inflated neurons. Except with respect to the general topography of the lesions these thus differ from those in FLD.

Other Pathology behind Disorders with Clinical Similarities to FLD

This group (table 4) contained 27 cases and was dominated by dementia of Alzheimer's type in 9 cases with either an extraordinary severity of the Alzheimer changes in the frontal cortex and/or severe frontal white matter incomplete infarction [6]. The next biggest group, 5 cases, showed a pure form of incomplete white matter infarction again with a frontal predominance, without cortical changes. Four cases had in addition complete infarctions in the shape of lacunes on the basis of hypertensive angiopathy and were diagnosed as Binswanger's disease with the common frontal predominance of the subcortical changes. In the last two groups subcortical lesions may have resulted in a frontal cortical disconnection syndrome. There were also two cases of trauma with widespread frontal white matter destruction but limited cortical lesions and 1 case of Jakob-Creutzfeldt's disease with frontally dominating cortical lesions. Most of these diagnoses were encountered also in the previous material with the addition of bilateral thalamic infarcts in one case.

Discussion

The recent material of 10 cases of FLD had a histopathological picture identical to that noted in the previous material of 16 cases. Three further cases (table 2) differ with respect to extent and severity of changes. These cases are accepted as a form of FLD, only more advanced than observed in our previous case material and those in table 1. The number of old and new neuropathologically verified cases of FLD thus amounts to 29 cases. They all have in common a consistent frontal or frontotemporal distribution of simple degenerative changes and the absence of Alzheimer or Pick changes and vascular abnormalities as well as Lewy bodies or indications of prion disease. The impression of a superficial, supragranular cortical affliction is fortified by the antiubiquitin and GFAP analysis showing positivity restricted to the superficial cortical layers. Cases in table 2 also add the impression that FLD may progress to a more advanced stage than experienced in the first study. The lack of antiprion antibody positivity and the negative results of molecular biological genetic studies underscore the unlikelihood of a prion etiology although more extensive studies would be needed for a safe statement. The overall picture also shows a mild to insignificant involvement of the basal ganglia, the thalamus and usually only mild involvement of the substantia nigra.

A consistent feature was the middle age debut of the disease and the relatively short duration entirely eliminates cases of this sort from material of dementia after age 80 [7]. Some other disorders with a clinical similarity to FLD due to a frontal mainpoint of changes considerably expand the clinical group of dementia of frontal type, especially those listed in table 4. In the literature there are several descriptions of a condition similar to FLD. Jagust et al. [8] reported a SPECT study on FLD patients, showing a hypoperfusion of both frontal lobes in contrast to the posterior hypoperfusion seen in Alzheimer's disease. Further analogies are hampered by a lack of neuropathology investigation in this report. Also Miller et al. [9] reported 8 cases with frontal lobe degeneration where SPECT revealed frontal and temporal hypoperfusion with relative preservation of parietal and occipital blood flow. Similar findings were reported by Kumar [10].

The combination of ALS and changes as in FLD have previously been reported [11–14] and lately by Neary et al. [15], where 4 patients showed the frontal lobe changes here reported. In a case of this kind, Ferrer et al. [16] reported the same findings and added reduced cortical neuronal dendritic arbors, proximal dendritic varicosities and depletion of dendritic spines as shown by rapid Golgi staining. This together with our findings of a reduced synaptic density through measurements of synaptophysin optical density [unpubl. results] may indicate a primary or early involvement of the synaptodendritic apparatus of the neurons in the superficial cortical layers which give rise to short association fibers. Massé et al. [17] have also described a case with similar pathology though with additional probably distinguishing features as deep cortical layer involvement and pronounced astrocytic gliosis of the white matter, thalamus and inferior olives bringing their case closer to progressive subcortical gliosis.

A pathology similar to that in FLD as described here was reported in some cases by Knopman et al. [18] under the name of dementia lacking distinctive histologic features. At variance with our findings was in additional cases a severe involvement of the hippocampus, the thalamus and substantia nigra. With regard to the widespread cortical involvement, however, there are similarities to our probable FLD cases listed in table 2.

Green et al. [19] reported on a case of progressive aphasia progressing to dementia, which on neuropathological examination showed changes similar to those reported here in FLD though more widespread than in the majority of our cases. A clinical course of this kind with a possible dissemination of cortical changes to wide areas may again indicate the possibility of a more focal start for the disease not only in the frontal lobes but in motor speech areas with later spread throughout the cortex, something that might be suspected to have happened in our probable FLD cases number 2–4 in table 2. Cases of this kind may be found among the patients with semantic dementia described by Snowden et al. [20] though histopathological confirmation is here lacking. A later report [21] lists 3 autopsy-studied cases of progressive language disorder with clinical and pathological similarities to FLD. Additional examples of dementia of frontal lobe type strikingly similar to FLD both from a clinical and a neuropathological point of view are on record [22, 23]. Also closely similar cases have been described in a large family [24]. Even with a rather cautious selection of cases from the literature FLD is thus evidently a rather widespread and not uncommon dementing disorder and may make up as much as 8–10% of organic dementias according to our study. At a time when dementia has become almost synonymous to Alzheimer's disease it is important to point out that there are thus other dementing disorders of importance, not only from a diagnostic point of view but also for the sake of purity of scientific materials for etiologic or therapeutic studies.

The consistency of structural and topographic changes in our cases can be taken to indicate a pathological entity. It is characterized by a basic primary degenerative process with loss of dendrites and synapses and, in the end, of neurons particularly of the associative superficial laminae in the frontal cortex with a secondary glial scarring and microvacuolation. FLD is therefore tentatively classified in a non-Alzheimer group with frontal disorders such as semantic or progressive dementia, some of the cases described in the literature as dementia lacking distinctive histology, Pick's disease and ALS with dementia.

Acknowledgements

Supported by grants from the Medical Faculty, Lund University, Lund, Sweden, the Swedish Medical Research Council, Greta Kock Johan Kock's Foundation, Svenska Alzheimer-föreningen.

Kerstin Sturesson and Annette Persson are gratefully acknowledged for their skilled histotechnical assistance.

References

1 Brun A: Frontal lobe degeneration of non-Alzheimer type. I. Neuropathology. Arch Gerontol Geriatr 1987;6:193–208.
2 Englund E, Brun A: Frontal lobe degeneration of non-Alzheimer type. IV White matter changes. Arch Gerontol Geriatr 1987;6:235–244.
3 Gustafson L: Frontal lobe degeneration of non-Alzheimer type. II Clinical picture and differential diagnosis. Arch Gerontol Geriatr 1987;6:209–223.
4 Risberg J: Frontal lobe degeneration of non-Alzheimer type. III Regional cerebral blood flow. Arch Gerontol Geriatr 1987;6:225–233.
5 Collinge J, Palmer M, Mahal S, Campbell T, Hardy J, Brown J, Brun A, Gustafson L, Backer B, Roos R: Absence of prion protein mutations in familial Pick's disease and dementia of frontal lobe type, in press.
6 Brun A, Englund E: A white matter disorder in dementia of the Alzheimer type: A pathoanatomical study. Ann Neurol 1986;19:253–262.
7 Brun A, Gustafson L, Samuelsson SM, Ericsson C: Neuropathology of late life. Dementia 1992;3:125–130.
8 Jagust W, Reed B, Seab P, Kramer J, Budinger T: Clinical-Physiologic Correlates of Alzheimer's Disease and Frontal Lobe Dementia. New York, Liss, 1989.
9 Miller BL, Cummings JL, Villanueva-Meyer J, Boone K, Mehringer CM, Lesser IM, Mena I: Frontal lobe degeneration: Clinical, neuropsychological, and SPECT characteristics. Neurology 1991;41:1374–1382.

10 Kumar A, Schapiro MB, Haxby JV, Grady CL, Friedland RP: Cerebral metabolic and cognitive studies in dementia with frontal behavioral features. J Psychiatr Res 1993, 97–109.
11 Hudson AJ: Amyotrophic lateral sclerosis and its association with dementia. Parkinsonism and other neurological disorders: A review. Brain 1981;104:217–247.
12 Morita K, Kaiya H, Ikeda T, Namba M: Presentile dementia combined with amyotrophy: A review of 34 Japanese cases. Arch Gerontol Geriatr 1987;6:263–277.
13 Wikström J, Paeteau A, Palo J, Sulkava R, Haltia M: Classic amyotrophic lateral sclerosis with dementia. Arch Neurol 1982;39:681–683.
14 Mitsuyama Y, Kogoh H, Ata K: Progressive dementia with motor neuron disease. Additional case report and neuropathological review of 20 cases in Japan. Eur Arch Psychiat Neurol Sci 1985;235:1–8.
15 Neary D, Snowden JS, Mann DMA, Northen B, Goulding PJ, MacDermott N: Frontal lobe dementia and motor neuron disease. J Neurol Neurosurg Psychiatry 1990;53:23–32.
16 Ferrer I, Roig C, Espino A, Peiro G, Matias Guiu X: Dementia of frontal lobe type and motor neuron disease. A Golgi study of the frontal cortex. J Neurol Psychiatry 1991;54: 932–934.
17 Massé G, Mikol J, Brion S: Atypical presenile dementia. Report of an anatomo-clinical case and review of the literature. J Neurol Sci 1981; 52:245–267.
18 Knopman DS, Mastri AR, Frey WH II, Sung JH, Rustan T: Dementia lacking distinctive histologic features: A common non-Alzheimer degenerative dementia. Neurology 1990;40: 251–256.
19 Green J, Morris JC, Sandson J, McKeel DW Jr, Miller JW: Progressive aphasia: A precursor of global dementia? Neurology 1990;40:423–429.
20 Snowden JS, Goulding PJ, Neary D: Semantic dementia: A form of circumscribed cerebral atrophy. Behav Neurol 1989;2:167–182.
21 Snowden JS, Neary D, Mann MA, Goulding PJ, Testa HJ: Progressive language disorder due to lobar atrophy. Ann Neurol 1992;31: 174–183.
22 Neary D, Snowden JS, Northen B, Goulding P: Dementia of frontal lobe type. J Neurol Neurosurg Psychiatr 1988;51:353–361.
23 Neary D, Snowden JS: Dementia of the frontal lobe type; in Levin HS, Eisenberg HM, Benton AL (eds): Frontal Lobe Function and Dysfunction. Oxford, Oxford University Press, 1991, pp 304–317.
24 Brown J, Gydesen S, Sorenson A, Brun A, Smith S, Houlden H, Twells R, Mullan M, Rossor M, Collinge J, Palmer M, Goate A, Hardy J: Genetic characterization of a familial non-specific dementia originating in Jutland, Denmark, in press.

Dementia 1993;4:132–136

David S. Knopman

Department of Neurology,
University of Minnesota Hospitals,
Minneapolis, Minn., USA

Overview of Dementia Lacking Distinctive Histology: Pathological Designation of a Progressive Dementia

Key Words
Dementia
Frontal lobes

Abstract
The group of progressive dementing illnesses that lack distinctive histologic features includes at least four variants: a cortical type, a thalamostriate type, a motor neuronopathy type and a leukogliotic type. While the clinical presentation of some cases is that of anterograde amnesia, progressive aphasia and dysexecutive syndrome are the most common initial symptom complexes. A large number of reported cases are familial, although no abnormal gene has been identified. Pathologically, these illnesses are defined by cortical, hippocampal, striatal, medial thalamic, nigral and motor nuclei cell dropout and astrogliosis. In some cases, white matter gliosis is striking. Identification of specific histological or molecular markers of at least some of these conditions will greatly advance our understanding of these specific conditions as well as dementing illnesses in general.

Introduction

Dementia lacking distinctive histology (DLDH) defines a group of dementing illnesses whose neuropathological presentation involves no distinctive subcellular dysmorphic features such as neurofibrillary tangles, Pick bodies, Lewy bodies or ballooned cells.

Several neuropathological subgroups can be identified based on the distribution of cell loss: cortical DLDH, thalamostriatal DLDH, and DLDH with motor neuronopathy. A dementing illness in which the white matter changes are most prominent – progressive subcortical gliosis – may also be included in this group. Although the DLDH group is heterogeneous, there are a number of common features, including early onset, rapid progression and positive family histories.

The prevalence of this group of diseases has varied greatly in different reports. In the dementia autopsy series of 460 cases from which Knopman et al. [1] drew their cases, it represented 3% of cases overall, but 10% of the under-age-70 group. In the Lund series of 158 dementia cases, Brun [2] found 10% of autopsied degenerative dementia cases with nonspecific pathology designated as frontal lobe degeneration of the non-Alzheimer type. In

David Knopman, MD
Department of Neurology
Box 295
University of Minnesota Hospitals
Minneapolis, MN 55455 (USA)

1013–7424/93/0044–0132
$2.75/0

the series of Constantinidis et al. [3] of 32 patients who were labeled as Pick's lobar atrophy, 12 had some degree of fronto-temporal lobar atrophy, but neither Pick bodies nor swollen chromatolytic neurons, while 10 had Pick-body-positive disease.

DLDH – Cortical

Prominent language difficulty has been present in many of the DLDH – cortical-type patients who have been described [4, 5]. The language deficits may occur in the presence of intact nonverbal executive functions.

The following patient [Knopman, unpubl.] presented with anomia. She was 60 years old when she developed difficulties in producing the names of family members and friends. Psychometric testing showed poor verbal performance but excellent executive and visuospatial functions. Her verbal learning performance was good. She died after a 12-year course. At autopsy, there was marked 'thinning of the cortical ribbon with neuronal loss, astrogliosis and coarse vacuolation of the second cortical layer'. The changes were bilateral, but worse on the left, and were most noticeable in the prefrontal and temporal lobes. Changes in the hippocampus were limited to severe neuronal loss in the CA1 segment. The amygdala was severely degenerated. There were neurofibrillary tangles in the CA2 region of the hippocampus, but they were present in no other region, and senile plaques were absent. There were no Pick bodies or ballooned cells.

Gustafson [6] described a frontal lobe degeneration of the non-Alzheimer type that may be identical to DLDH with cortical involvement. This condition presents in a nonaphasic manner that may be dominated by marked changes in behavior: 'restless, aggressive, hypersexual, unrestrained und unreliable'. A second patient was a first cousin of the first. She presented as 'euphoric, disinhibited ... and forgetful ... She also showed dyscalculia and expressive dysphasia'. The clinical presentation was notable for 'changes and dissolution of personality, behavior and speech, rather than ... cognitive deterioration'.

Several of the patients in the series of Neary et al. [7] with 'dementia of the frontal lobe type' probably also fall into the category DLDH-cortical. These patients presented with 'social misconduct and personality change, unconcern and disinhibition ...' Neuropsychologically, they demonstrated inattention, impaired memory, generally preserved spatial abilities, and sparse spontaneous speech. Almost half of the cases of Neary et al. had a positive family history of dementia.

The family reported by Kim et al. [8] probably also fits into the category of DLDH-cortical.

The prototypical pathology seen in DLDH-cortical includes prominent cortical cell loss throughout the frontal and temporal neocortex, and to a lesser extent, parietal cortex. Astrogliosis of the affected gray matter structures invariably accompanied the neuronal loss. Subcortical nuclear regions may be affected but to a mild degree.

DLDH – Thalamostriatal

A second neuropathological subgroup of DLDH is one in which cell loss and astrogliosis are prominent in multiple subcortical regions but especially in the thalamus and striatum. The heterogeneity of the neuropathology makes generalizations about this group difficult. Indeed, some of the cases have had predominantly striatal involvement [9–12], while others have had mainly thalamic involvement [13, 14]. In other cases, both regions were involved [1, 11].

The clinical presentation of DLDH-corticostriate patients is one in which new learning deficits plus elements of dysexecutive syndrome occur. Behavioral aberrations – manifestations of the disinhibition and poor judgement of the dysexecutive syndrome – have stood out in the reported patients.

Torack and Morris [10] described a 57-year-old woman who presented with irritability and social withdrawal. She was oriented, but had 'pressured speech, poor comprehension, poor recent and remote memory and impaired insight'. She showed increased interest in sexual matters, and engaged in uncharacteristic behaviors. She died after a 7-year illness. The brain showed prominent cell loss in substantia nigra, caudate nucleus, amygdala, orbital-frontal cortex, subiculum and parahippocampal cortex. There was prominent white matter gliosis only in the regions underlying the orbital cortex. These authors emphasized that the distribution of the neuropathological changes followed a pattern consistent with the nonstriatal dopaminergic pathways, in light of the prominence of the medial nigral damage.

Six of the cases in Knopman et al. [1] had prominent thalamostriatal involvement in addition to the cortical and nigral changes. In these cases both thalamic and striatal cell loss were prominent. Their cognitive deficits led to the initial diagnosis, but later, motor system deficits occurred. For example, patient 3 [1] developed memory loss and a change in personality at age 46 years. He forgot the names of fellow workers and disregarded job responsibilities. He became belligerent with his wife and shoved her on one occasion and swore at her, behaviors that were absent from this man's premorbid disposition. A CT scan showed caudate atrophy. Later in the course of his illness, grunting and then anarthria occurred. He died 9 years after the onset of the first symptoms. Neuropathologically, the frontal and temporal cortex changes were identical to those described above. Hippocampal and amygdalar changes were also similar. In addition, though, there was severe cell loss in the putamen, caudate nucleus, medial thalamus and substantia nigra. The neuropathological changes in the cases reported by Knopman et al. [1] were very similar to those seen by Torack and Morris [10].

As with the DLDH-cortical cases, in the DLDH-thalamostriate type, one sees cortical involvement consisting of astrogliosis and cell loss with vacuolatio of upper cortical layers of frontal and temporal cortex. Gliosis of underlying white matter is mild. Some cases [13] will show motor neuron dropout, similar to DLDH-motor neuronopathy cases.

DLDH with Motor Neuronopathy

A third neuropathological subgroup of DLDH had cell loss and astrogliosis in cortical and subcortical cell groups and prominent cell loss in motor nuclei of the brainstem and spinal cord [1, 15–18]. More cases of this group have been reported than of the other DLDH subtypes.

The typical clinical history is that of cognitive impairment or dysphagia as the presenting symptom, relatively rapidly followed by the other. The duration of the illness has been between 2 and 7 years [1, 15–18], with those with shorter courses predominating. The presence of fasciculations, frank somatic muscle atrophy and prominent bulbar palsy has allowed some cases to be identified antemortem.

For example, patient 9 of Knopman et al. [1] presented at age 49 years with increasing difficulties in carrying out her daily activities. She ceased meal preparations, her personal hygiene and her housework deteriorated, and she became unable to deal with financial matters. She demonstrated the dysexecutive syndrome on neuropsychological testing. Although her new learning was impaired, she retained 50% of items in both verbal and nonverbal memory tests after a delay. One year later, she had become mute. She had had symptoms for 5 years at the time of death.

The pathology has been relatively consistent across reported cases. Cell loss has been mild to moderate in the frontal and temporal cortices. Sponginess of the upper cortical layers has usually been present. The sites of major cell loss have included the hippocampal formation, substantia nigra and the motor neurons of the hypoglossal nucleus. The anterior horn cells of the spinal cord have shown reduction in numbers, when the cord was available for examination [16]. Involvement of the striatum and thalamus has been modest, with some exceptions [13]. Dopaminergic deficiency in the striatum was a prominent finding in several patients [15, 18], with normal cholinergic function [1, 15, 18].

DLDH with Leukogliosis (Progressive Subcortical Gliosis)

Subcortical gliosis should be considered along with the other forms of DLDH since its clinical presentation is similar, and there is some overlap in its neuropathological expression.

Most of the reported cases have been between 30 and 60 years old at onset [19–21]. Illness duration is highly variable. Expressive speech difficulty or global cognitive impairment with marked personality changes occur at onset. The prominence of the cognitive changes and the absence of typical neurological findings of white matter pathway involvement suggests that progressive subcortical gliosis is less like multiple sclerosis and more like a gray matter degeneration. Some cases may be familial [19].

The brain in subcortical gliosis shows mild cortical and subcortical cell loss. The gliosis may be prominent in the gray matter, but it is very intense in white matter. There is usually minimal demyelination. In Neumann and Cohn's cases [19], additional neuropathological findings besides the marked astrocytosis in subcortical white matter included marked neuronal loss in the caudate, thalamus, insula, midbrain tectum and tegmentum, inferior olives and some cortical regions, especially the cingulate gyrus. In Verity and Wechsler's cases [21] the subcortical gray matter changes were also present, but variable in location: thalamic in their first case, and striatal in the second case.

The prominence of the white matter gliotic process is the major point of difference between progressive subcortical gliosis, as the term is used here, and DLDH-thalamostriatal type. Otherwise, the subcortical gray matter neuronal loss and astrogliosis of this condition appear highly overlapping with DLDH-thalamostriate.

Clinical Diagnostic Challenges of the Non-Alzheimer Dementias

The best time to diagnose DLDH cases is when the distinctive patterns of cognitive dysfunction are present, early in the course of the patient's symptoms. Later, as patients become progressively more impaired, the differences between Alzheimer's disease and DLDH become lost in the global cognitive decline that is likely to be evident.

Some of our cases of DLDH have presented with mainly anterograde amnesia, making them virtually indistinguishable from AD. In the majority of cases, however, the early stages of the DLDH cases exhibit patterns other than global dysfunction or anterograde amnesia. One such pattern is nonfluent aphasia. The syndrome of progressive aphasia without dementia [4] includes DLDH cases.

The other distinctive pattern of cognitive dysfunction that occurs in the DLDH group is one in which a dysexecutive syndrome is prominent. In addition to direct frontal lobe involvement, damage to subcortical structures that are reciprocally connected with the frontal lobes such as the caudate nuclei or the medial dorsal thalamic nucleus may produce the dysexecutive syndrome. The latter regions are sometimes involved in DLDH cases.

Although the cognitive dysfunction of DLDH cases overlaps sufficiently with AD to preclude the development of highly precise differentiation from AD, it is possible to suspect them based on the types of presentations described above.

The Neuropathological Uncertainties of the Non-Alzheimer Dementias

By definition, the cases reported under the label of DLDH lack specific macroscopic or microscopic neuropathological features. Does frontotemporal atrophy confer any commonality in pathogenesis to these diseases? Transsynaptic effects of subcortical projection pathway diseases (e.g., the nonstriatal dopaminergic pathway [10]) might link the DLDH cases, but more evidence is needed.

The presence of spongiform changes is nonspecific also. Is it merely a result of the gliotic process, or does it too confer specificity? The obvious association raised by the spongiform change is that these diseases might be related to prion disease. We have sequenced the prion gene in several of our patients and found a deletion of one of the octapeptide repeats in one patient [22], but no protease-resistant prion protein was detected in the brain of this patient. While it is likely that this deletion represents a nonpathological polymorphism, it is possible that it could predispose to brain degeneration. In 4 other patients, including one family with several members of one generation affected, no sequence changes were present in the prion gene. We are continuing to examine this issue in additional patients.

The degree of subcortical neuronal loss is quite variable across all of the diseases discussed, ranging from negligible noncerebral cortical changes to multisystem involvement as well as anterior horn cell loss. Are these subcortical neuronal changes the key to diagnosis or are they incidental to the cortical disease?

Finally, the degree of subcortical white matter pathology is also quite variable. The entity progressive subcortical gliosis specifically involves white matter disease as a dominant finding. To what extent is axonal loss or demyelination at the core of the other diseases, or is it all a secondary loss?

Ultimately, we must learn more about the underlying molecular mechanisms of these diseases to answer these various questions. Increased clinical recognition and increased interest in the neuropathology of these disorders should see a movement beyond phenomenological definitions and on the molecular definitions of these diseases.

References

1 Knopman DS, Mastri AR, Frey WH II, Sung JH, Rustan T: Dementia lacking distinctive histologic features: A common non-Alzheimer degenerative dementia. Neurology 1990;40:251–256.

2 Brun A: Frontal lobe degeneration of non-Alzheimer type. I. Neuropathology. Arch Gerontol Geriatr 1987;6:193–208.

3 Constantinidis J, Richard J, Tissot R: Pick's disease: Histological and clinical correlation. Eur Neurol 1974;11:208–217.

4 Kirshner HS, Tanridag O, Thurman L, Whetsell WO Jr: Progressive aphasia without dementia: Two cases with focal spongiform degeneration. Ann Neurol 1987;22:527–532.

5 Mehler MF, Horoupian DS, Davies P, Dickson D: Reduced somatostatin-like immunoreactivity in cerebral cortex in nonfamilial dysphasic dementia. Neurology 1987;37:1448–1453.

6 Gustafson L: Frontal lobe degeneration of non-Alzheimer type. II. Clinical picture and differential diagnosis. Arch Gerontol Geriatr 1987;6:209–223.

7 Neary D, Snowden JS, Northen B, Goulding P: Dementia of frontal lobe type. J Neurol Neurosurg Psychiatry 1988;51:353–361.

8 Kim R, Collins G, Parisi J, Wright A, Chu Y: Familial dementia of adult onset with pathological findings of a nonspecific nature. Brain 1981;104:61–78.

9 Adams RD, Van Bogaert L, Vander Eecken H: Striato-nigral degeneration. J Neuropathol Exp Neurol 1964;23:584–608.

10 Torack RM, Morris JC: Mesolimbocortical dementia. A clinicopathological case study of a putative disorder. Arch Neurol 1986;43:1074–1078.

11 Moossy J, Martinez AJ, Hanin I, Rao G, Yonas H, Boller F: Thalamic and subcortical gliosis with dementia. Arch Neurol 1987;44:510–513.

12 Verity MA, Roitberg B, Kepes JJ: Mesolimbocortical dementia: Clinicopathological studies on two cases. J Neurol Neurosurg Psychiatry 1990;53:492–495.

13 Deymeer F, Smith TW, DeGirolami U, Drachman DA: Thalamic dementia and motor neuron disease. Neurology 1989;39:58–61.

14 Little BW, Brown PW, Rodgers-Johnson P, Perl DP, Gajdusek DC: Familial myoclonic dementia masquerading as Creutzfeldt-Jakob disease. Ann Neurol 1986;20:231–239.

15 Horoupian DS, Thal L, Katzman R, Terry RD, Davies P, Hirano A, et al: Dementia and motor neuron disease: Morphometric, biochemical, and Golgi studies. Ann Neurol 1984;16:305–313.

16 Neary D, Snowden JS, Mann DMA, Northen B, Goulding PJ, Macdermott N: Frontal lobe dementia and motor neuron disease. J Neurol Neurosurg Psychiatry 1990;53:23–32.

17 Wikstrom J, Paetau A, Palo J, Sulkava R, Haltia M: Classic amyotrophic lateral sclerosis with dementia. Arch Neurol 1982;39:681–683.

18 Gilbert JJ, Kish SJ, Chang LJ, Morito C, Shannak K, Hornykiewicz O: Dementia, parkinsonism, and motor neuron disease: Neurochemical and neuropathological correlates. Ann Neurol 1988;24:688–691.

19 Neumann MA, Cohn R: Progressive subcortical gliosis, a rare form of presenile dementia. Brain 1967;90:405–418.

20 Masse G, Mikol J, Brion S: Atypical presenile dementia: Report of an anatomo-clinical case and review of the literature. J Neurol Sci 1987;52:245–267.

21 Verity MA, Wechsler AF: Progressive subcortical gliosis of Neumann: a clinicopathologic study of two cases with review. Arch Gerontol Geriatr 1987;6:245–261.

22 Diedrich JF, Knopman DS, List JF et al: Deletion in the prion protein gene in a demented patient. Hum Mol Genet 1992;1:443–444.

Dementia 1993;4:137–142

Yoshio Mitsuyama

Department of Psychiatry, Miyazaki Medical College, Miyazaki, Japan

Presenile Dementia with Motor Neuron Disease

Key Words
Presenile dementia
Motor neuron disease

Abstract
Seventy-one Japanese cases of presenile dementia with motor neuron disease were reviewed. The clinico-pathological features were: (1) progressive dementia with insidious onset, mostly in the presenile period: (2) neurogenic muscular wasting in the course of illness (ALS- or SPMA-like symptoms); (3) duration from the onset of the illness to death: 2–5 years (average 30.6 months); (4) extrapyramidal symptoms and definite sensory deficits are less commonly present; (5) no characteristic abnormalities in the CSF or EEG; (6) no known consanguinity or familial occurrence; (7) non-specific mild to moderate degenerative changes in the fronto-temporal cerebral cortex, hypoglossal nuclei and spinal cord, and frequently in the substantia nigra. The author was interested in discovering whether the frequency and topology of lesions in the brain of patients with presenile dementia and motor neeuron disease differed characteristically from the distribution found in cases of Alzheimer's disease, Pick's disease, Creutzfeldt-Jakob disease or progressive subcortical gliosis. Presenile dementia with motor neuron disease might be a new disease entity.

Introduction

Presenile dementia with motor neuron disease has been described by the author in 1979 [1] and 1984 [2] as a new clinico-pathological entity. Increasing numbers of such patients have been recognized since that time and the development of single-photon emission tomography (SPECT) using radioactive tracer (^{123}I-IMP-SPECT) has made it possible to provide and objective correlate of the purported frontal abnormalities.

Methods and Result

Seventy-one similar cases of presenile dementia with motor neuron disease have been reported in Japan between 1964 and 1992 [3] (table 1). The average age of onset was 58.6 (38–74) years for females and 53.5 (40–75) years for males (table 2). The mean age for sexes combined was 55.4 years. The duration of illness of both sexes was 30.6 (10–72) months on the average. The male/female sex ratio was 1.7. The author has classified the patients into typical and atypical cases according to their clinico-pathological characteristics shown in table 3. Both types are included in the same disease entity with a common pathogenesis. Patients showed progressive dementia with insidious onset, mostly in the presenile period. The psychiatric symptoms in cases of presenile dementia with motor neuron disease are shown in table 4. They consisted of memory difficulty, global intellectual impairment, personality change, emotional disorders and loss of spontaneous speech. These symptoms were usually interpreted as unclassified presenile dementia. They were not typical of Alzheimer's or Pick's disease in their clinical

Yoshio Mitsuyama, MD
Department of Psychiatry
Miyazaki Medical College
5200 Kihara, Kiyotake
Miyazaki, 889-16 (Japan)

1013–7424/93/0044–0137
$2.75/0

course. Reduction of speech seemed to be more characteristic in the early stage of the illness and the disease usually did not develop into a severely deteriorated state even in an advanced stage of the disease. Personality change also was mild to slight and personal contact preserved fairly well. There were some differences in the psychiatric symptoms between Pick's disease and presenile dementia with motor neuron disease. No apraxia or agnosia, which frequently is seen in Alzheimer's disease, was found in any case.

Neurological symptoms in cases of presenile dementia with motor neuron disease are shown in table 5. Neurogenic muscle atrophy, bulbar symptoms (dysphagia, dysarthria), and occasional pyramidal signs were included. Patients have been diagnosed as having amyotrophic lateral sclerosis or spinal progressive muscular atrophy. Neurological symptoms usually developed 6–12 months after the onset of psychiatric symptoms, but some cases showed neurological symptoms before the appearance of psychiatric symptoms, and in others the symptoms appeared almost simultaneously. Neurogenic muscle atrophy was seen in all of the cases and muscular wasting was prominent in the distal portion of the upper extremities, shoulder and face (fig. 1). The legs were less involved and patients could walk steadily even in the terminal stage. Bulbar symptoms became evident in the stage of muscle atrophy and were progressive, causing death. Pyramidal signs such as increased deep tendon reflexes and Babinski signs were rarely observed. Extrapyramidal signs such as rigidity, tremor and myoclonic jerk-

Table 1. Cases of presenile dementia with motor neuron disease (MND) in Japan (clinical and autopsied cases in 1964 – 1992; n = 71) [3]

	Typical cases (n = 53)	Atypical cases (n = 18)
Male:female	35:18	10:8
Age at onset, years	54.2 (38–69)	58.8 (40–75)
Age at death, years	57.3 (39–70)	60.5 (43–80)
Initial symptoms		
Dementia, %	43.3	55.6
MND, %	18.9	22.2
Dementia + MND, %	37.7	22.2
Interval between dementia and neurology, months	10.4 (3–24)	29.0 (4–64)

Table 2. Presenile dementia with motor neuron disease in Japan (1964–1992) (death cases: n = 58) [3]

	Age at onset years	Age at death years	Duration months
Female (n = 19)	58.6 (38–74)	60.4 (39–80)	29.6 (10–72)
Male (n = 39)	53.5 (40–75)	56.9 (43–77)	30.8 (12–72)
Total (n = 58)	55.4 (38–75)	58.1 (39–80)	30.6 (12–72)

Table 3. Clinico-pathological classification of presenile dementia with motor neuron disease (MND)

	Typical	Atypical
Onset	presenile	presenile to senile
Dementia	slight to moderate	slight to severe
Neurology	MND	MND
	no ophthalmoplegic signs	occasional ophthalmoplegic signs (PSP-like)
	less pyramidal signs	often pyramidal signs
Interval between dementia and neurology	within 12 months	after 24 months
Neuropathology	frontal > temporal	temporal > frontal
	cortical, cortico-nigral degeneration	subcortical gliosis
	no senility changes	often senility changes

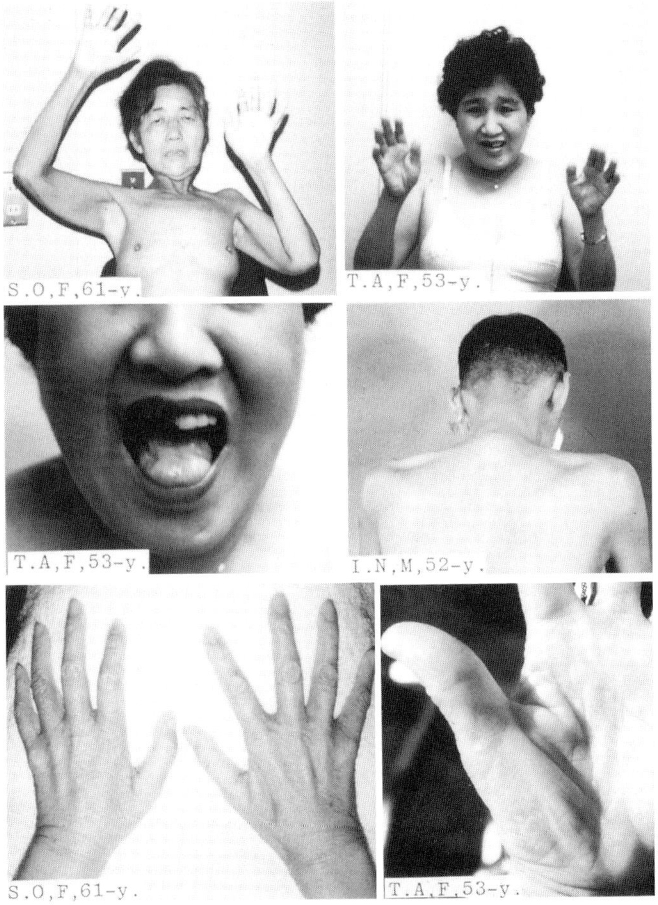

Fig. 1. Muscle atrophy and weakness of the upper extremities, tongue, shoulder and thenar muscle.

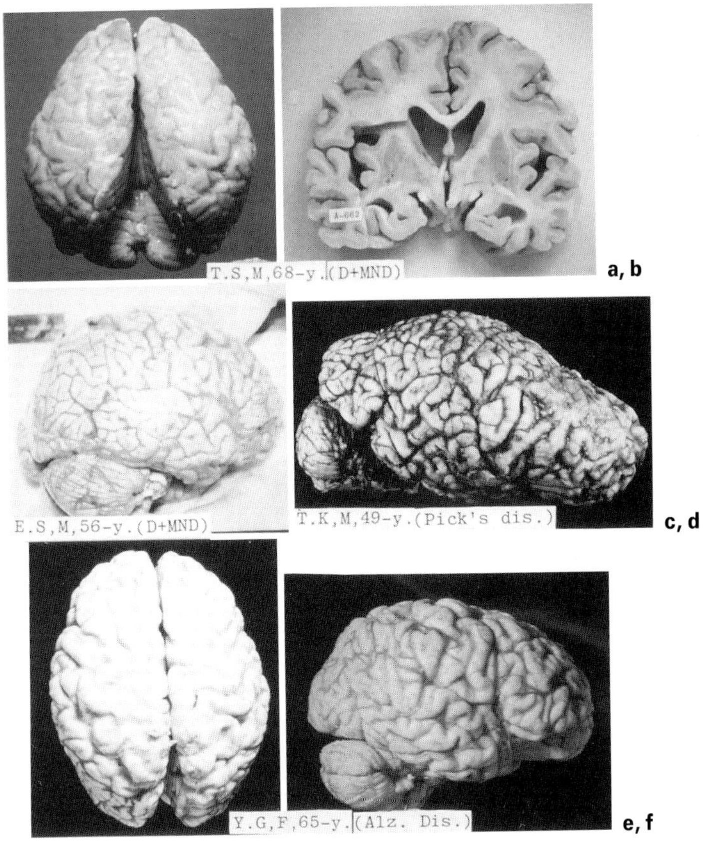

Fig. 2. Macroscopic findings of the brains in presenile dementia with motor neuron disease (**a–c**) compared with Pick's disease (**d**) and Alzheimer's disease (**e, f**).

Table 4. Psychiatric symptoms in cases of presenile dementia with motor neuron disease

	Typical cases (n = 53)	Atypical cases (n = 18)
Memory loss, %	100	100
Cognitive impairment, %	100	100
Affective disorders, %	83	78
Personality disorders, %	85	72
Reduced activity, %	81	58
Progressive aphasia, %	49	22
Uncontrolled behavior, %	57	50
Stehende Redensart, %	21	11
Perseveration, %	12	0
Echolalia, %	7	0
Delusion, delirium halucination, %	6	11

Table 5. Neurological symptoms in cases of presenile dementia with motor neuron disease

	Typical cases (n = 53)	Atypical cases (n = 18)
Neurogenic muscle atrophy, %	100	100
Dysarthria, dysphagia, %	86	83
Pyramidal sign (Babinski's sign), %	16	40
Hand tremor, %	9	6
Masklike face, %	2	6
Rigidity, %	4	12
Hypersalivation, %	2	0
Myoclonus, %	2	0
Supranuclear ophthalmoplegia, %	0	28
Urinary incontinence, %	2	12
Primitive reflex, %	2	0

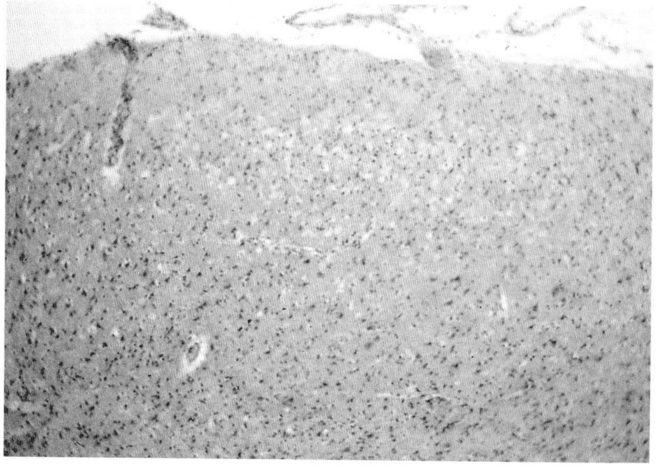

3

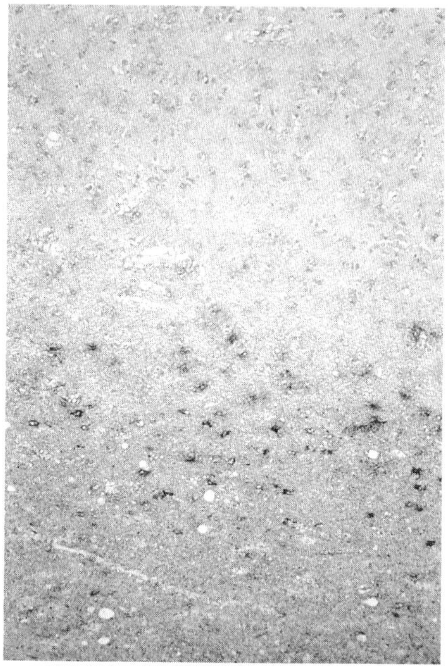

4

Fig. 3. Status spongiosus in the superficial layers of the superior frontal gyrus. HE. ×300.

Fig. 4. Subcortical gliosis in the superior frontal gyrus. GFAP. ×225.

Table 6. Neuropathology of cases of presenile dementia with motor neuron disease in Japan

	Typical cases (n = 32)	Atypical cases (n = 15)
Average brain weight, g	1,235 (1,000–1,470)	1,207 (1,090–1,340)
Brain atrophy		
Frontal, %	56	27
Fronto-temporal, %	41	33
Temporal, %	3	40
Cortical neuronal loss, %	100	100
Neurogenic muscle atrophy, %	100	100
Anterior horn cell loss, %	100	100
Loss of hypoglossal nuclei, %	88	67
Sponginess in cerebral cortex, %	66	33
Subcortical gliosis, %	81	87
Neuronal loss and gliosis in substantia nigra, %	59	47
Cortico-spinal tract degeneration, %	38	33
Loss of Betz's cell, %	16	7
Buina body, %	22	20
Senile plaques, NFT, granulovacuolar degeneration, %	0	60

ing were also rarely observed. Patients did not develop generalized rigidity or spasticity in their clinical courses.

Fourty-seven or 71 cases of presenile dementia with motor neuron disease which were reviewed had pathological studies of the brain and spinal cord. General pathology showed bronchopneumonia as an immediate cause of death in all cases. Gross inspection of the brain (fig. 2) in the majority of these cases showed atrophy that varied from slight to moderate, mainly in the frontal and/or temporal lobes. The principal neuropathological findings are shown in table 6. Nonspecific neuronal degeneration, characterized by mild to slight disappearance of neurons and simple atrophy in the cerebral cortex, coexisted with lesions similar to those seen in motor neuron disease such as neurogenic muscle atrophy. The lesions in the cerebral cortex were predominant in layers 2 and 3 in the frontal and temporal regions. Mild to slight spongy appearance of the cortex was present in the 2nd and 3rd layers (fig. 3). Fibrillary astrogliosis in the subcortical white matter of the cerebral hemisphere was frequently observed with variable severity from case to case (fig. 4). Lesions in the spinal cord and hypoglossal nuclei were more commonly found (fig. 5–7). Senile plaques, Alzheimer's neurofibrillary tangles and granulovacuolar degeneration were not found in the typical cases but were frequently present in the atypical cases with late onset after 60 years. Although some of the patients showed pyramidal tract degenera-

5
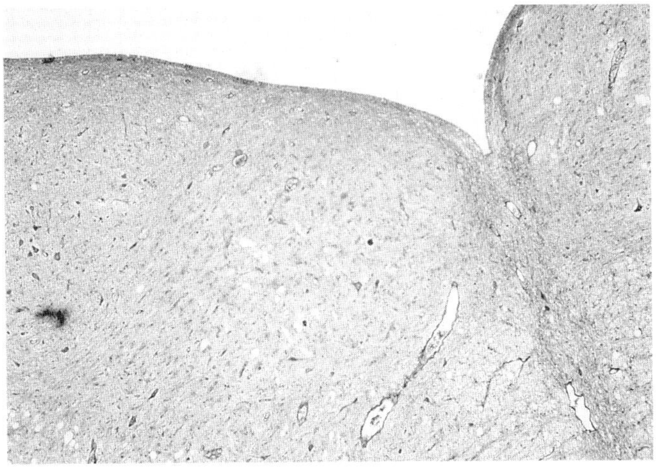

7
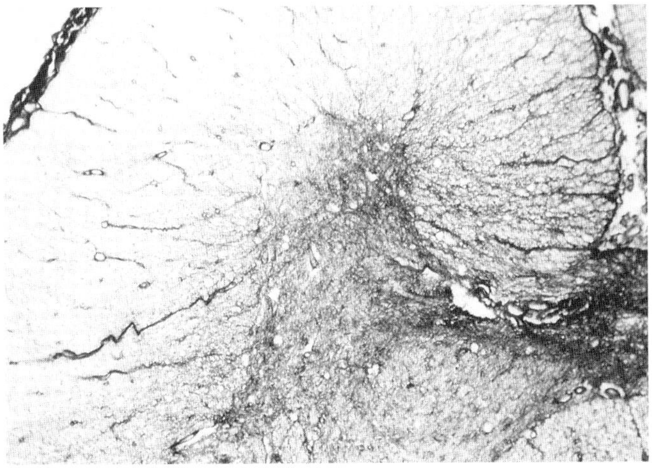

6

8
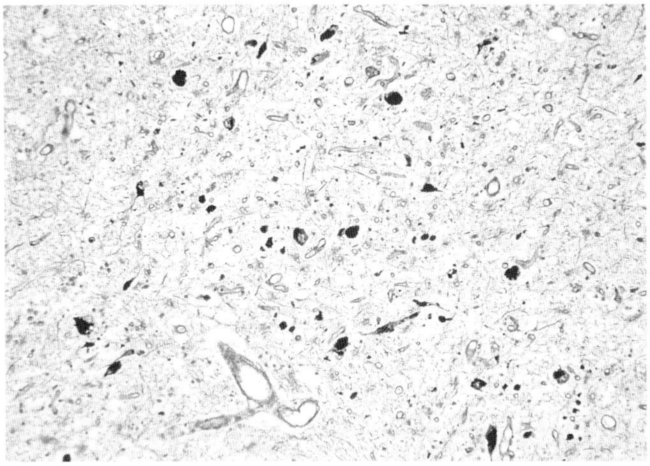

Fig. 5. Neuronal loss and gliosis of hypoglossal nuclei. Bodian. ×120.

Fig. 6. Neuronal loss of anterior horn cell in the cervical spinal cord. HE. ×120.

Fig. 7. Gliosis in the gray matter of the cervical spinal cord. Holzer. ×120.

Fig. 8. Depigmentation and gliosis in the substantia nigra. HE. ×300.

tion, it was very mild compared with that seen in the classical sporadic amyotrophic lateral sclerosis. Degeneration of the substantia nigra or globus pallidus was frequently observed (fig. 8). There was no case with cerebrovascular lesions caused by arteriosclerotic vessel disease.

Discussion

The term 'presenile' may not be appropriate to describe some patients who developed dementia after the age of 65. No localized areas with increased incidence have been observed in Japan and there is no geographical preference since we find similar cases in such countries as Germany [4, 5], France [6, 7], North America [8–10] and Finland [11].

The clinico-pathological criteria of presenile dementia with motor neuron disease described by the author are as follows; (1) frontal-type progressive dementia with insidious onset, mostly in the presenile period; (2) neurogenic muscular wasting in the course of illness (ALS- or SPMA-like symptoms); (3) duration from illness to death: 2–5 years (average 30.6 months); (4) extrapyramidal symptoms and definite sensory deficits are less commonly present; (5) no characteristic abnormalities in the CSF or EEG; (6) no known parental consanguinity or familial occurrence; (7) nonspecific mild to moderate degenerative changes in the fronto-temporal cerebral cortex, hypoglossal nuclei and spinal cord, and frequently in the substantia nigra.

From the epidemiological point of view, presenile dementia with motor neuron disease is similar to classical sporadic amyotrophic lateral sclerosis and the clinical features resemble those of other known primary degenerative dementias such as Alzheimer's disease, Pick's disease, progressive subcortical gliosis and Creutzfeldt-Jakob disease. However, selective cognitive dysfunction, language impairment such as logoclonia and visuo-spatial disorientation that are frequently seen in Alzheimer's disease were not observed in any case of presenile dementia with motor neuron disease. 'Stehende Redensarten' that are frequently observed in Pick's disease were seen in several cases of presenile dementia with motor neuron disease. Neuro-radiological studies in all these cases showed fronto-temporal atrophy, and psychiatric symptoms were suggestive of Pick's disease rather than Alzheimer's disease. Advanced dementia has not been reported in classical sporadic amyotrophic lateral sclerosis, and amyotrophic lateral sclerosis-like symptoms usually have not been described in classical Alzheimer's or Pick's disease.

In the cases of presenile dementia with motor neuron disease, there were usually no definite pyramidal signs or pathological reflexes and the distribution pattern of muscular atrophy was not identical to that found in classical sporadic amyotrophic lateral sclerosis. Muscular weakness and wasting have been described early in the course of Pick's disease and during the terminal phase of Alzheimer's disease [2]. The amyotrophic form of Creutzfeldt-Jakob disease is clinically indistinguishable from these cases of presenile dementia with motor neuron disease.

The pathological findings in these cases of presenile dementia with motor neuron disease were essentially similar. Neuronal loss and degeneration characterized by simple atrophy and mild to slight status spongiosus in the upper layers were the main pathological features in the cortex. They were not consistent with those of Alzheimer's disease or Pick's disease, and clinico-pathological information allowed no other definitive diagnosis. Lesions in the brain stem and spinal cord were very different from those in progressive subcortical gliosis. It has been reported that the presence of Alzheimer's neurofibrillary tangles in the hippocampus and substantia nigra is a paramount finding in Guamanian amyotrophic lateral sclerosis and Parkinsonism-dementia complex of Guam [5, 10]. Although some authors [9, 11] observed that dementia is part of the amyotrophic lateral sclerosis syndrome from the review of amyotrophic lateral sclerosis-dementia case reports, pathological studies of the central nervous system in presenile dementia with motor neuron disease showed a low incidence of loss of Betz's cell and pyramidal tract degeneration. It is proposed that amyotrophic lateral sclerosis syndrome is part of the same process as primary degenerative dementia from its clinico-pathological appearance and may be one of the disorders making up a larger group where frontal lobe degeneration may be one component. The similarity of their clinical manifestations and pathological findings at autopsy has suggested that presenile dementia with motor neuron disease could be a single disease rather than a variant of amyotrophic lateral sclerosis or Creutzfeldt-Jakob disease.

References

1 Mitsuyama Y, Takamiya S: Presenile dementia with motor neuron disease. Arch Neurol 1979; 36:592–593.

2 Mitsuyama Y: Presenile dementia with motor neuron disease in Japan: Clinico-pathological review of 26 cases. J Neurol Neurosurg Psychiatry 1984;47:953–959.

3 Hirano A, Malamud E, Elizan TS, Kurland LK: Amyotrophic lateral sclerosis and parkinsonism-dementia complex on Guam. Further pathologic studies. Arch Neurol 1966;15:35–51.

4 Minauf M, Jellinger K: Kombination von amyotrophischer Lateralsklerose mit Pickscher Krankheit. Arch Psychiatr Nervenkr 1969;212: 279–288.

5 von Poppe W, Tennstedt A: Klinische und pathologisch-anatomische Untersuchungen über Kombinationsformen praeseniler Hirnatrophien (Pick, Alzheimer) mit spinalen atrophisierenden Prozessen. Psychiatr Neurol 1964;145:322–344.

6 Bonduelle M: Amyotrophic lateral scerosis; in Vinken PJ, Bruyn GW (eds): Handbook of Clinical Neurology. Amsterdam, North-Holland, 1975, vol 22, pp 281–338.

7 Brion S, Psimaras A, Chevalier JF, Plas J, Massa G, Jatteau O: L'association maladie de Pick et sclérose latérale amyotraphique. Encéphale 1980;6:259–286.

8 Horoupian DS, Thal L, Katzman R, Terry RD, Davis P, Hirano A, DeJeresa R, Fuld PA, Petito C, Blass J, Ellis JM: Dementia and motor neuron disease: Morphometric, biochemical and Golgi studies. Ann Neurol 1984;16: 305–313.

9 Hudson AJ: Amyotrophic lateral sclerosis and its association with dementia, parkinsonism and other neurological disorders. A review. Brain 1981;104:217–247.

10 Myrianthopoulos NC, Smith JK: Amyotrophic lateral sclerosis with progressive dementia. Neurology 1962;12:603–610.

11 Wickstrom J, Pateau A, Palo J, Sulkava R, Halita M: Classic amyotrophic lateral sclerosis with dementia. Arch Neurol 1982;39:681–683.

Dementia 1993;4:143–148

Lars Gustafson

Department of Psychogeriatrics, Lund, Sweden

Clinical Picture of Frontal Lobe Degeneration of Non-Alzheimer Type

Key Words
Frontal lobe degeneration of non-Alzheimer type
Frontal lobe dementia
Pick's disease
Regional cerebral blood flow
Neuropathological diagnoses

Abstract
Frontal lobe degeneration of non-Alzheimer type (FLD) is the second most common primary degenerative dementia in southern Sweden. Clinical findings in 30 FLD cases with postmortem-verified diagnoses are described. FLD starts in the presenium with a mean disease duration of 7.5 years (range 3–17 years). Clinical onset is insidious and slow and the early stage is dominated by personality changes with lack of insight and judgement and signs of disinhibition. A typical feature is progressive loss of expressive speech with stereotyped phrases, late mutism and amimia. Restlessness, changes of oral/dietary behavior and utilization behavior are prevalent as also psychotic features. Temporal and spatial orientation are usually preserved for a long time in contrast to Alzheimer's disease. Dementia in FLD is similar to that of Pick's disease and ALS with dementia. Early recognition of FLD seems possible based on standardized clinical evaluation supported by neuropsychological tests, measurement of regional cerebral blood flow and other types of brain imaging. The etiology of FLD is unknown but a positive heredity was reported in 60%.

This paper focuses upon clinical aspects of frontal lobe degeneration of non-Alzheimer type (FLD) and the possibility of differentiating it from other organic and non-organic mental diseases on clinical grounds. FLD is a new clinico-pathological entity although there is no reason to believe that the disease is new. It has existed for generations and so have the clinical questions it raises. The first observations on the relationship between localized frontal or fronto-temporal cortical atrophy in dementia and symptoms of aphasia was published 100 years ago by Pick [1]. His findings were followed up by further pathological and clinical evidence of a disease entity, Pick's disease, different from the presenile dementia described by Alzheimer [2]. The emphasis of dementia research on Alzheimer's disease (AD) during the last decades has been rewarding although possibly contributing to some neglect of other less common degenerative dementias.

Why this great interest in FLD in Lund and a few other places? Is FLD for some reason linked to certain populations or geographic regions? This might be the case, but probably there are other reasons for the comparatively large number of FLD patients in our catchment area. One important factor might be the selection criteria of patients in the longitudinal dementia study that started 25 years ago [3]. The patients in this study were referred to the psychiatric department and since 1984 to the psychogeriatric department because of symptoms of dementia. Moreover, during the first 5 years only patients with presenile dementia were selected. The clinical repertoire was designed for differential diagnosis of dementia and espe-

Lars Gustafson
Department of Psychogeriatrics
PO Box 638
S-220 09 Lund (Sweden)

1013–7424/93/0044–0143
$2.75/0

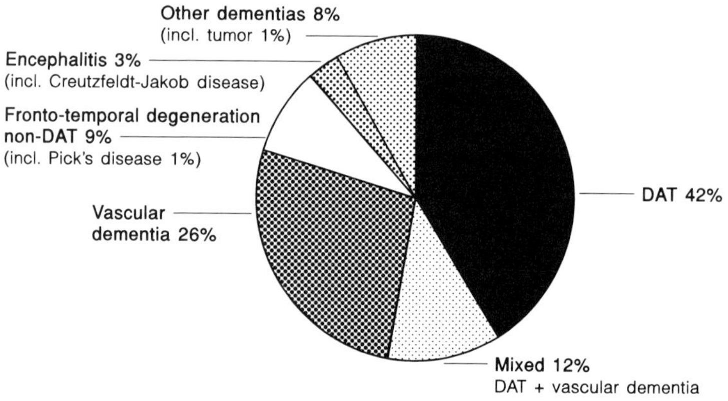

Fig. 1. Causes of organic dementia. Neuropathological diagnoses in 400 patients. Lund longitudinal study 1992. DAT = Dementia, Alzheimer type.

cially for recognition of treatable organic brain syndromes as pseudodementia due to non-organic mental diseases. This approach revealed the clinical and diagnostic heterogeneity of dementia conditions. Three out of the first 10 patients happened to display an organic frontal lobe pattern with lack of judgement, disinhibition and emotional changes, but dysgnosia and dyspraxia were only present in one case. The significance of these findings was supported by regional cerebral blood flow (rCBF) measurements showing blood flow decreases in frontal areas. rCBF measurements with the ^{133}Xe clearance technique were performed from the start of the longitudinal study [4]. The non-traumatic xenon inhalation technique has been available since 1975. At present, it is performed with a 254 detector high-resolution (Cortexplorer) equipment [5]. Functional brain imaging thus made it possible to reveal general, focal, symmetrical and asymmetrical flow abnormalities in dementia and to relate these findings to the clinical manifestations. Until the neuropathological findings in deceased cases were revealed [6, 7], the tentative clinical diagnosis in patients with frontal lobe features had been Pick's disease.

The neuropathological diagnosis in the first 150 deceased cases was AD in about 50% and AD in combination with vascular brain damage in an additional 10%. However, this patient sample dominated by early-onset dementia also contained 16 cases with FLD and 4 cases with Pick's disease. This material was presented at the first meeting on FLD in Lund 1986 and published a year later [8]. The designation FLD was suggested after great hesitation to indicate its pathological and clinical differences from the majority of cases with AD. In our most recent survey of 400 cases (fig. 1), FLD was found in 8% and Pick's disease in 1% of the total material. These results possibly indicate the importance of the patient's age at onset of dementia which was higher in this extended patient material.

Other research groups have been working with similar clinical material. Neary et al. [9], in Manchester, have reported a large study of 26 patients with presenile-onset 'dementia of frontal lobe type' in 1988. Single-photon computerized tomography (SPECT) indicated anterior brain damage in all patients. There was a striking similarity between the clinical picture in these cases and our findings. Neary [10] has suggested that dementia of frontal lobe type may be responsible for as much as 20% of early-onset dementia.

Clark et al. [11] found 22 cases with primary degenerative dementia without Alzheimer pathology in a consecutive series of deceased cases. The majority of these cases showed frontal and/or temporal cortical atrophy. The pathological diagnosis was Pick's disease in 6 cases and non-specific degeneration in 7 cases. Thus non-Alzheimer frontal lobe pathology was common also in this material. In 1990, Knopman et al. [12] presented 14 cases with 'dementia lacking distinctive histology' among 460 dementia cases referred to a brain bank. These patients with frontal and temporal or parietal degeneration of non-Alzheimer and non-Pick type comprised 10% of the patients below 70 years of age compared to Pick's disease found in 6.8%. The detailed clinical description of cases with dementia lacking distinctive histology indicates that many of them fall within the same clinical frames as our FLD cases. This material has been further presented at this congress [13].

Table 1. Clinical characteristics in FLD, Pick's disease and AD

	FLD (n = 30)	Pick's disease (n = 6)	AD (n = 21)
Sex M/F	14/16	0/6	4/17
Age at onset, years	54.2 ± 7.8 (35–70)	51.2 ± 11.1 (35–65)	57 ± 5 (45–65)
Age at death, years	61.8 ± 8.3 (41–77)	60.2 ± 13.4 (42–72)	67 ± 5 (56–75)
Duration, years	7.6 ± 3.6 (3–17)	9 ± 5.3 (4–17)	10.6 ± 3 (5–16)
Heredity for dementia, %	60	50	30

The relationship between FLD and Pick's disease still remains an open question. The vast literature on Pick's disease has in many ways touched upon clinical and pathological questions regarding FLD in a wider sense. In 1974, Constantinides et al. [14] described a 'typical Pick material' with lobar atrophy without neuronal swellings or argyrophilic inclusions and a clinical picture with moria, bipolar mood changes, bulimia, echolalia and stereotyped activities similar to those of our FLD material. With our rather limited experience of Pick's disease, it has not been possible, however, to differentiate the two diseases clinically. The difference has to be confirmed with neuropathological examination and genetic evidence. To my knowledge, FLD and Pick's disease have not been diagnosed in the same family.

This presentation of clinical findings in FLD is based on data from 30 cases (16 old and 14 new) with postmortem-verified diagnoses. I will also consider observations in patients who have been followed for many years until death but lacking the postmortem investigation. The clinical diagnoses were strongly supported by rCBF and neuroradiological findings.

The first symptoms of FLD start in the presenium although in occasional cases somewhat later. The mean duration of the disease is 7.5 years with a wide range from 3 to 17 years. The sex distribution is equal, and positive heredity of dementia of similar type was recorded in 60%. These background data are very similar to what has been reported in our previous study and in accordance with other studies [6, 8] (table 1).

The clinical onset is usually slow and insidious. The early stage is dominated by deterioration of personality, behaviour and speech. The cognitive impairment is less obvious although memory failure and lack of concentration are present. Surprisingly, often dyscalculia is mentioned as an early impairment. Temporal and spatial orientation are usually preserved for a long time although often difficult to evaluate by traditional methods (table 2).

Table 2. Clinical findings in FLD

- Insidious onset and slow progression
- Changes of personality
  - Disinhibition, social neglect
  - Levelling of emotions
  - Lack of insight and judgement
  - Irritability, restlessness
  - Anxiety, euphoria
  - Apathy
- Dissolution of language
  - Progressively reduced speech
  - Stereotyped phrases
  - Echolalia
  - Mutism, amimia
- Depressive episodes
- Hypochondriasis, pain
- Deceptions, delusions
- Changes of oral/dietary behaviour
- Sterotype behaviour
- Memory, receptive speech and spatial functions comparatively spared
- Dyscalculia
- Intermittent dyspraxia
- Epileptic seizures less common
- Syncopal attacks

The personality changes may stand out as rather unspecific and therefore often difficult to interpret as expressions of organic brain disease. Even close relatives may have difficulties to decide when the first symptom appeared and the duration of the disease may easily be underestimated. Signs of disinhibition, lack of judgement, restlessness and irritability are found early in FLD. The impaired control and modulation of emotions are seen as tearfulness, inadequate smiling and spells of crying, later developing to hypomimia.

There is a general levelling of emotions with lack of empathy and insight into ill health. The patient becomes self-centred, less concerned about his family and friends. The emotional tuning may be that of euphoria, sometimes combined with confabulation and increased talkativeness. True Witzelsucht (pathological punning) is however rare in our material. The emotional changes may sometimes be difficult to differentiate from a hypomanic or manic state. Differential diagnosis against major depression may also be difficult, since FLD patients may have episodes of depressed mood with suicidal thoughts. The patient's apathy, social withdrawal, hypomimia and reduced speech may also be misinterpreted as a non-organic depression.

The patient's emotional changes and unpredictable behaviour may lead to confrontations with and even rejection from the family and society. The disinhibition may lead to acts of violence, offensive behaviour, shoplifting and increased alcohol consumption. An important consequence of the diagnostic process is the opportunity to offer understanding of a patient's strange behaviour and strategies to handle the situation. It is important to alleviate the pressure on the family by psychological and social support and when necessary to offer hospital care for diagnosis and treatment.

Restlessness and an irresistible impulse to explore the environment are often observed. This 'utilization behaviour' has been described in patients with focal frontal lobe lesions [15] and resembles the 'metamorphosis' of the Klüver-Bucy syndrome in animals. Other components of this syndrome in man such as disinhibited oral behaviour with excessive smoking, drinking and eating and preference of special food and reduced emotions are also prevalent in FLD.

The disease may also lead to traffic accidents. The patient becomes inattentive and careless, exceeds speed limits and neglects traffic lights. The patient may fully agree that his driving has changed but does not consider this as strange or indicating a disease. The typical Alzheimer patient is more self-critical an anxiously aware of his difficulties to handle a car. Their left-right insecurity is easily revealed since most elderly learned driving before 1967, when Sweden changed from left to right hand traffic.

Most FLD patients deny any awareness of a mental disease and see very little reason for a medical examination. However, several patients display various somatic complaints often symptoms of pain and bizarre hypochondriasis [9]. These patients may frequently demand medical examinations because of the somatic symptoms.

Psychotic symptoms, such as hallucinations and illusions have been described in all types of dementia although the frequencies vary markedly between different studies. In our longitudinal study, hallucinations and illusions were reported in about 25% of patients with FLD or Pick's disease, in 25% of AD with early onset and in 50% of late-onset AD. The psychotic symptoms in FLD show a high variability [16] and the combination with other frontal lobe traits such as lack of insight, disinhibition, restlessness and communication difficulties makes it difficult to handle these patients with psychological techniques. The clinical picture might easily be misinterpreted and a tentative clinical diagnosis was often schizophrenia at an early stage. The association between psychosis and frontal lobe damage has also been described in vascular dementia and in AD with degeneration and ischemic white matter lesions in the frontal lobes [17, 18].

A typical feature of FLD is a progressive loss of expressive speech which in Pick's disease has been described as 'dissolution du langage' or 'Sprachverödung' [19, 20]. It usually starts as a verbal aspontaneity with amnesic dysphasia, stereotyped comments with frequent repetitions of limited phrases. Imitating behaviour especially echolalia was recorded in about 50% of our cases. The writing may also change in various ways such as magnitude, misspellings and stereotypes. These changes are different from the dysgraphia in AD. The symptom constellation of palilalia, echolalia, mutism and amimia the s.c. PEMA syndrome of Guiraud [21] is typical of FLD and Pick's disease and rare in AD.

All our patients developed general cognitive deterioration before death although with somewhat varying severity. Patients with progressive dysphasia as described by Snowden et al. [22], Mesulam [23] and others do not necessarily develop dementia although generalized cognitive impairment usually of frontal lobe type eventually develops in many cases.

There were very few pathological somatic findings in our autopsy-verified FLD cases. A relatively high frequency of syncopal attacks has been reported in Pick's disease and therefore our observations of low mean blood pressure and a tendency to orthostatic blood pressure drop in FLD may be of special interest [24]. Neurological symptoms such as fascicular twitchings, muscular wasting, dysarthria, dysphagia and extrapyramidal signs may develop in patients with FLD as also described in Pick's disease. It might be difficult to differentiate FLD with a rapid course from Creutzfeldt-Jacob disease with frontal emphasis and ALS with dementia of frontal type. Neary [10] has reported several cases of rapidly progressive dementia and motoneuron disease with a striking clinical and pathological similarity to FLD, and we have so far seen 4 FLD cases with neurological symptoms of this type. These questions are further analysed in this volume

[25]. The association between FLD and ALS with frontal lobe dementia is further indicated by a high frequency of normal EEG and fronto-temporal atrophy on brain imaging in both types of dementia.

There are several significant differences between FLD and AD, especially concerning symptoms at an early stage of the disease. Memory failures, spatial disorientation and to some extent dyspraxia is more frequent in AD while lack of insight, disinhibition and changes of oral dietary behaviour is more prevalent in FLD [8]. Language disturbances also differ. Stereotyped speech, echolalia and mutism combined with preserved receptive speech are typical for FLD while global dysphasia, logoclonia, increased muscular tension and epileptic seizures are more common in AD. EEG is usually normal at an early stage of FLD but almost always pathological in AD [26, 27]. A diagnostic problem might be that a minority, about 5%, of Alzheimer cases show a frontal lobe predominance of degeneration and clinic. These patients show, in addition to symptoms of AD such as dysphasia, dyspraxia and dysgnosia, also early personality changes with emotional lability, euphoria, inadequate laughing and loss of insight [17]. It is important to consider the total clinical picture and brain-imaging findings for these patients to reach a correct ante mortem clinical diagnosis.

The differential diagnosis between early FLD and Huntington's disease may also be critical when personality changes and psychotic features dominate. However, CT scan and MRI may reveal a gradual loss of the heads of the caudate nuclei and PET may be an early predictor of the development of Huntington's disease. Different types of vascular dementia may also be mistaken for FLD clinically. Several cases with selective incomplete white matter infarctions in the frontal lobes displayed a mainly psychiatric symptomatology and the clinical diagnosis of FLD was sometimes considered. These patients showed personality changes with disinhibition, spells of anxiety and aggressiveness, language dysfunction and in some cases hallucinations and delusions [17]. There are also patients with slowly developing Binswanger's disease with a clinical picture dominated by emotional lability with periods of euphoria, apathy or depression while disinhibition and loss of insight were rather uncommon [17]. A frontal lobe clinic was also observed in multi-infarct dementia with frontal emphasis and in patients with strategic subcortical infarcts such as bilateral thalamic infarcts [7].

Early recognition of FLD (and Pick's disease) seems possible based on a standardized clinical evaluation supported by neuropsychological testing, brain imaging and other diagnostic techniques. We use a combination of three diagnostic rating scales; one for diagnosis of AD [29], one for recognition of FLD [29] and the ischemic score developed by Hachinski [30] to estimate the possibility of a vascular dementia. The scoring procedure offers a check on the quality of the clinical information. Diagnoses based on the scoring profile in the three rating scales have been validated against rCBF and neuropathological findings [31]. My last point is that the clinical diagnosis of dementia condition should be encouraged and guided by the diagnostic classifications. DSM III-R [32] and ICD-10 [33] do not, however, facilitate recognition and classification of organic dementia with frontal features. So far only the Swedish consensus on ante mortem classification of dementia seems to have taken the importance of FLD into consideration [34, 35].

Acknowledgements

The present study was supported by the Swedish Medical Research Council (grant 3950), the Greta and Johan Kock Foundation and the Medical Faculty, Lund University.

I gratefully acknowledge Anette Welin for secretarial help.

References

1 Pick A: Über die Beziehungen der senilen Hirnatrophie zur Aphasie. Prager Med Wochenschr 1892;17:165–167.

2 Alzheimer A: Über eine eigenartige Erkrankung der Hirnrinde. Neurol Centrabl 1907;18: 177–179.

3 Gustafson L, Hagberg B: Dementia with onset in the presenile period. A cross-sectional study. Acta Psychiatr Scand 1975;suppl 257:9–71.

4 Ingvar DH, Gustafson L: Regional cerebral blood flow in organic dementia with early onset. Acta Neurol Scand 1970;suppl 46:42–73.

5 Risberg J, Gustafson L, Brun A: High resolution regional cerebral blood flow measurements; in Maurer K, Riederer P, Beckman H (eds): Alzheimer's Disease. Epidemiology, Neuropathology, Neurochmistry, and Clinics. Wien, Springer, 1991, pp. 357–364.

6 Brun A: Frontal lobe degeneration of non-Alzheimer type. I. Neuropathology. Arch Gerontol Geriatr 1987;6:193–208.

7 Brun A: Frontal lobe degeneration of non-Alzheimer type revisited. Dementia 1993;4:126–131.

8 Gustafson L: Frontal lobe degeneration of non-Alzheimer type. II. Clinical picture and differential diagnosis. Arch Gerontol Geriatr 1987;6: 209–223.

9 Neary D, Snowden JS, Northen B, Gouldin P: Dementia of frontal lobe type. J Neurol Neurosurg Psychiatry 1988;51:353–361.
10 Neary D: Dementia of frontal lobe type. J Am Geriatr Soc 1990;38:71–72.
11 Clark AW, White III CL, Manz HJ, et al: Primary degenerative dementia without Alzheimer pathology. Can J Neurol Sci 1986;13: 462–470.
12 Knopman DS, Mastri AR, Frey WH, et al: Dementia lacking distinctive histologic features: A common non-Alzheimer degenerative dementia. Neurology 1990;40:251–256.
13 Knopman D: Overview of dementia lacking distinctive histology: pathological designation of a progressive dementia. Dementia 1993;4: 132–136.
14 Constantinidis J, Richard J, Tissot R: Pick's disease. Histological and clinical correlations. Eur Neurol 1974;11:208–217.
15 Lhermitte F, Pillon B, Serdaru M: Human autonomy and the frontal lobes. I. Imitation and utilization behavior: A neuropsychological study of 75 patients. Ann Neurol 1986;19:326–334.
16 Gustafson L, Risberg J: Deceptions and delusions in Alzheimer's disease and frontal lobe dementia; in Levy R, Katona C, Levy R (eds): Delusions and hallucinations in old age. London, Gaskell, 1992.
17 Brun A, Gustafson L: Psychopathology and frontal lobe involvement in organic dementia; in Iqbal K, McLachlan DRC, Winblad B, et al (eds): Alzheimer's disease: Basic Mechanism, Diagnosis and Therapeutic Strategies. London, Wiley, 1991, pp 27–33.
18 Miller BL, Cummings JL, Villanueva-Meyer J, et al: Frontal lobe degeneration: Clinical, neuropsychological, and SPECT characteristics. Neurology 1991;42:1374–1382.
19 Delay J, Neveu P, Desclaux P: Les dissolutions du langage dans la maladie de Pick. Rev Neurol 1944;76:37–38.
20 Van Mansvelt J: Pick's disease. A syndrome of lobar, cerebral atrophy; its clinicoanatomical and histopathological types; thesis, Utrecht, 1954.
21 Escourolle R: La maladie de Pick. Etude critique d'ensemble et synthèse anatomo-clinique. Paris, Foulon, 1958.
22 Snowden JS, Neary D, Mann MA, Goulding PJ, Testa HJ: Progressive language disorder due to lobar atrophy. Ann Neurol 1991;31: 174–183.
23 Mesulam MM: Slowly progressive aphasia without generalized dementia. Ann Neurol 1982;11:592–598.
24 Warkentin S, Passant U, Minthon L, Karlson S, Edvinsson L, Fäldt R, Gustafson L, Risberg J: Redistribution of blood flow in the cerebral cortex of normal subjects during head-up postural change. Clin Auton Res 1992;2:119–124.
25 Mitsuyama Y: Presenile dementia with motorneuron disease. Dementia 1993;4:137–142.
26 Johannesson G, Brun A, Gustafson L, Ingvar DH: EEG in presenile dementia related to cerebral blood flow and autopsy findings. Acta Neurol Scand 1977;56:89–103.
27 Rosén I, Gustafson L, Risberg J: Multichannel EEG frequency analysis and somatosensory evoked potentials in patients with different types of organic dementia, accepted for publication.
28 Risberg J, Passant U, Warkentin S, Gustafson L: Regional cerebral blood flow in frontal lobe dementia of non-Alzheimer type, accepted for publication.
29 Gustafson L, Nilsson L: Differential diagnosis of presenile dementia on clinical grounds. Acta Psychiat Scand 1982;65:194–209.
30 Hachinski VC, Iliff LD, Zilhka E, du Boulay GH, McAllister VL, Marshall J, Ross Russell RW, Symon L: Cerebral blood flow in dementia. Arch Neurol 1975;32:632–637.
31 Risberg J, Gustafson L: Regional cerebral blood flow in psychiatric disorders, in Knezevic S, Maximilian VA, Mubrin Z, Prohovnik I, Wade J (eds): Regional cerebral blood flow. Lawrence Erlbaum, Hillsdale, 1988, pp 219–240.
32 American Psychiatric Association: DSM-III-R: Diagnostic and statistical manual of mental disorders, ed 3, revised. Washington, American Psychiatric Press, 1987.
33 World Health Organization: Tenth revision of the International Classification of Disease (ICD-10). 1988 draft of chapter V. Geneva, WHO, 1988.
34 Wallin A: Vascular dementia – pathogenetic and clinical aspects; thesis, Göteborg, 1989.
35 Gustafson L: Clinical classification of dementia conditions. Acta Neurol Scand 1992; suppl 139:16–20.

Dementia 1993;4:149–153

D. Frank Benson

Department of Neurology,
UCLA School of Medicine,
Los Angeles, Calif., USA

Progressive Frontal Dysfunction

Key Words
Frontal dementia
Frontal systems
Supramodal association cortex

Abstract
A number of causes of progressive mental impairment show a preponderance of frontal lobe symptoms. It is proposed that these disorders can be subdivided into primary and secondary frontal dementias, based on the symptomatology and the site of major pathological disruption. An anatomical explanation, based on variations in cortical and subcortical influences, aids in understanding the clinical differences.

Broadly defined, dementia is an acquired intellectual impairment sufficient to interfere with vocational or social activities [1]. While routinely viewed as a diffuse, general or global aberration of brain function, almost no clinical examples of dementia conform to such a broad, inclusive description. On the other hand, truly focal dementias that involve only a limited brain area or a specific function are relatively rare. Pick's disease is the single well-established example of focal degenerative dementia, but this disorder is infrequently noted in the clinic [2] and has traditionally proved difficult to diagnose. In the past decade, several additional brain disorders producing focal progressive impairments of cortical function have been demonstrated; examples include progressive aphasia [3, 4], posterior cortical atrophy [5] and frontal degenerative dementia [6, 7]. Following the initial demonstration only a few years ago, a surprisingly large number of different frontal degenerative disorders have been described [8–15]. They vary in both clinical and pathological characteristics to a degree sufficient to warrant categorization.

Several degenerative conditions producing structural, functional or clinical alteration of the frontal lobes resemble the clinical descriptions presented by Swedish investigators for frontal lobe degeneration of the non-Alzheimer type [6, 16]. Table 1 presents disorders with this clinical picture. All show microscopic pathological alterations that involve the frontal cortex; they will be classed as primary frontal degenerative dementias (table 1).

Table 1. Primary frontal degenerative dementia

Frontal lobe degeneration of the non-Alzheimer type
Frontal onset – Alzheimer's disease
Pick's disease
Progressive subcortical gliosis
Frontal onset – Jakob-Creutzfeldt disease

In addition to the primary disorders, a significant number of degenerative brain processes causing dementia produce frontal-type symptomatology but have a major pathological breakdown that involves subcortical or basal areas; these can be termed secondary frontal degenerative dementias (table 2). Both groups produce behavioral dysfunctions of the type usually related to frontal lobe abnormality but both clincial and pathological differences can be observed. A division into cortical and subcortical, as proposed by Cummings and Benson [17] for all dementias, appears both reasonable and correct.

D. Frank Benson
Department of Neurology
UCLA School of Medicine
710 Westwood Plaza
Los Angeles, CA 90024-1769 (USA)

1013–7424/93/0044–0149
$2.75/0

Table 2. Secondary frontal degenerative dementia

Movement disorders	
	Huntington's disease
	Progressive supranuclear palsy
	Parkinson's disease
	Cerebellar ataxia
	Multisystem atrophy
Vascular dementia	
	Lacunar disorder
	Binswanger's disease
Motor neurone disease	
Chronic alcoholism	
Neurosyphilis	
Thalamic infarction	

Table 3. Progressive frontal dysfunction: clinical variants

Characteristic	Primary	Secondary
Language defect	+++	+
Speech defect	+	+++
Motor function defect	+	+++
Reiterations, stereotypies	+++	+
Psychomotor retardation	+	+++
Disinhibition	+++	+
Klüver-Bucy symptoms	+++	+
Mood alteration (depression)	+	+++
Psychotic symptomatology		
Hallucinations	+	+++
Delusions	+++	+

+ = Mild abnormality; +++ = significant abnormality.

Clinical Distinctions

Foremost among the clinical findings indicating frontal degeneration is a significant alteration of interpersonal behavior. The alteration may take considerably different forms, ranging from severe apathy (abulia) and chronic depression to a euphoric, disinhibited agitation. The secondary frontal dementias tend to produce both motor and mental slowing, apathy and depression while the group listed as primary frontal dementias more often show disinhibited, restless and agitated behaviors. In both groups, the onset is insidious and the behavior pattern inconsistent. Language disorder, particularly difficulty in word-finding, is considerably more prominent in the primary frontal degenerations while speech problems such as hypophonia, dysarthria and dysprosody are often distinguishing features of the secondary group. Serial tests of memory and cognition reveal progressive decline in both groups, and visuospatial skills eventually become dilapidated in both. Striking exceptions may be seen in the last three response categories, however; some individuals with severe, disabling frontal-type behavior retain some or all competency in learning new material, in performing cognitive manipulations and/or carrying out visually oriented constructional tasks. In fact, partial or total retention of these skills in an otherwise behaviorally altered individual provides strong suggestion of a frontal disorder.

One obvious diagnostic distinction separating the primary from the secondary frontal degenerative disorders concerns the presence of motor abnormality. Many, but not all, disease processes that produce secondary frontal dysfunction show a prominent movement disorder. In some (e.g., motor neuron disease, Huntington's disease), the abnormal movements are diagnostic in themselves. In others (e.g., chronic alcoholism, vascular dementia), the motor findings may be relatively subtle. The presence of abnormal stance, gait or movements in a patient whose mentation, speech and behavioral responses have slowed suggests subcortical involvement. Depression, often of a significant degree, frequently accompanies the psychomotor retardation; the combination of personality change with slow mentation, abnormal movements and depression is often considered a frontal system disorder.

A number of notable behavioral findings are prominent in some cases of primary frontal dementia. The presence of Klüver-Bucy symptomatology (e.g., altered dietary preference, increased sexuality, decreased fear), a tendency to reiterate in conversation and to develop stereotyped mannerisms suggest primary frontal degeneration. Lack of social graces and restraints, poor judgment, tendency to flare with anger and grandiose or paranoid thinking may occur in both groups but the problems tend to be more distinct in the primary group. Hallucinations are relatively common in some of the secondary frontal disorders, whereas delusions are more suggestive of primary frontal degeneration. Table 3 compares selected behavioral features of primary and secondary degenerative frontal disorders.

Many other dementing disturbances, based on primary pathology elsewhere in the cerebrum, can produce frontal-type behavior along with other cognitive and neurological abnormalities. To clarify the position of the frontal lobes in the overall symptom picture of dementia, analysis of the basic functions of relevant cortical and subcortical processes is indicated.

Four Levels of Cortical Function

Based on clinical/anatomical correlations developed over the past century, four distinctly different types of neural function can be suggested for the human cortex. The four divisions represent levels of higher mental processing of progressive complexity, and can be termed primary, unimodal, heteromodal and supramodal. Each occupies a relatively specific anatomical locus and each appears to have distinct operational characteristics. Figure 1 shows a crude representation of the four types of cortex devoted to sensorimotor responses (limbic cortex is not discussed).

Primary sensory (and motor) cortex refers to the brain areas that receive stimuli from external sources (and Brodmann area 4, the primary motor cortex). The primary regions are relatively small, precisely defined cortical regions dedicated to processing basic stimuli in a single modality. The only cortical connections available to primary cortex are with adjacent unimodal association cortex and to homologous areas of primary cortex in the opposite hemisphere. The sole function of primary cortex is the reception and transfer of stimuli to adjacent neural aggregates of the same modality for additional, more sophisticated processing.

Unimodal association cortex, as the name implies, signifies association cortex that serves only a single modality. The four major modalities – visual, auditory, somesthetic and kinetic – each command a sizeable area of cortex. Smaller sensory systems (taste and smell) and limbic systems occupy more limited cortical territory and may not conform to the scheme presented here. In each unimodal system, primary stimuli are processed in the primary receptive area and then, through multiple interconnected synapses within that system's association cortex, subjected to additional, progressively more complex processing. The product of this operation is a *unimodal sensory percept*. Unlike the primary cortex, neurons of the unimodal association cortex have numerous connections to cells in heteromodal association cortex where unimodal sensory percepts can be further processed.

The third level of cortical function, *heteromodal association cortex* [18] acts as the neuronal core through which complex cognitive networks are developed. A rich matrix of connections across modalities becomes available

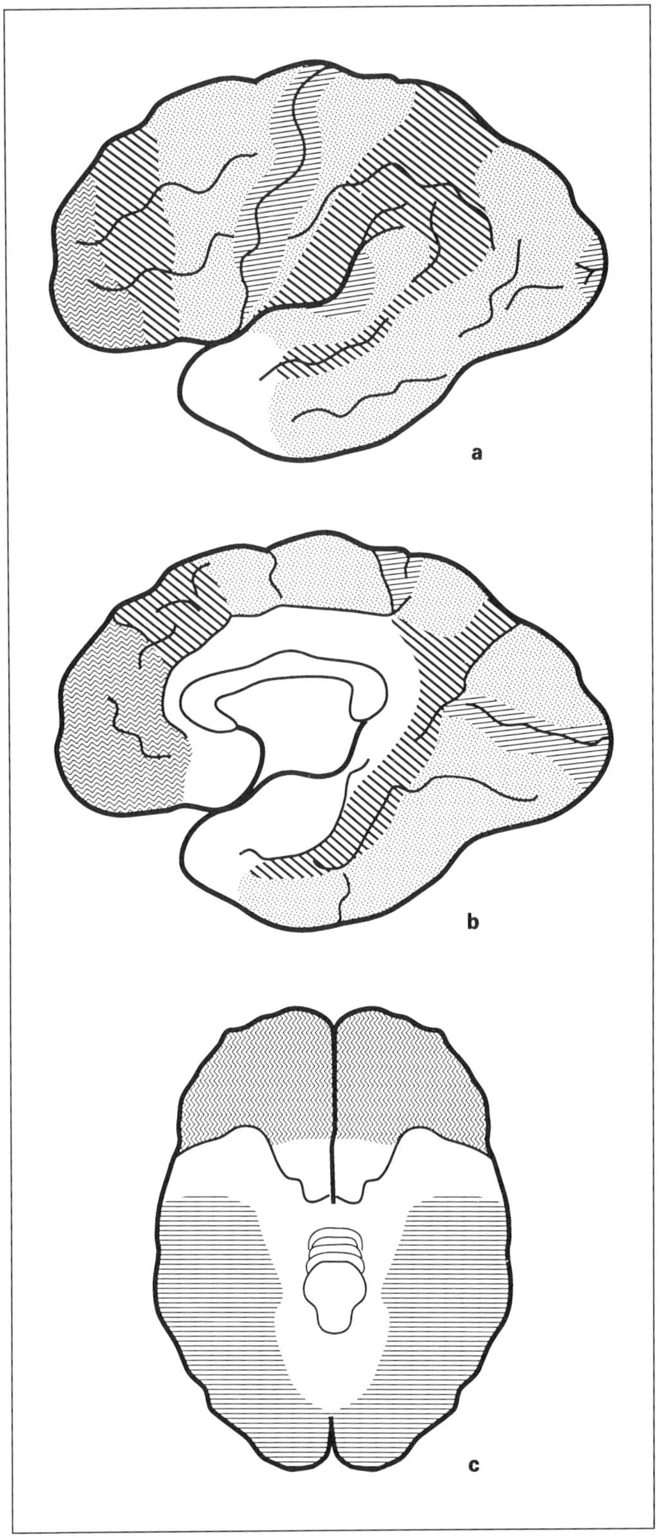

Fig. 1. Three diagrammatic views of cortex: (**a** lateral; **b** sagittal; **c** inferior) with four areas of cortex delineated (primary (isotypical) cortex = light horizontal lines; unimodal association cortex = dotted matrix; heteromodal association cortex = heavy diagonal lines; supramodal association cortex = horizontal wavy bands).

Table 4. Subcortical systems with prominent frontal connections

Reticular activating system
Limbic-hypothalamic system
Adrenal-pituitary axis system
Basal neurotransmitter system
Thalamic projection system
Basal ganglia/extrapyramidal system

through the heteromodal association cortex. Many names have been given to these areas (secondary, polymodal, cross-modal, multimodal, transmodal, heteromodal), most of which reflect the fact that associations are carried out across modalities. Unimodal percepts are intermixed, correlated with other percepts (primarily from memory stores) and integrated to produce complex psychological accomplishments such as language, constructional processing and cognitive manipulation. The extensive networks that carry out these functions include neurons and connections of both the heteromodal and the unimodal association cortices. Most information (memory) is stored within these cognitive networks and is accessed through multiple points within the neural complexes formed through the heteromodal association cortex. In addition, most cross-modal cognitive functions demand maintenance of serially presented material, at least over a short time span, a process defined as working memory [19, 20], temporal gradient [21] or sequencing [22]. The neural area most often considered essential for sequence maintenance is the dorsal convexity of the prefrontal cortex, an area that should be classed as heteromodal association cortex.

A fourth functional level, *supramodal association cortex*, includes some of the phylogenetically most recent regions of the prefrontal cortex and appears to operate as a monitoring system for the cognitive networks. Through ability to facilitate or inhibit the level of activity of individual cognitive networks, the supramodal association cortex exerts a powerful executive control over brain functions [23]. Management of the many simultaneously occurring activities of the heteromodal networks provides selective attention, anticipation, rumination, preplanning, response monitoring, future planning, self-analysis and other highest-level mental activities for human thought processing. Supramodal association cortex acts upon and controls, through selective inhibition, the activities of the vast number of cognitive networks constantly activated through the heteromodal and unimodal association cortices.

Each of the four levels of cortical activity is relatively distinct anatomically but the boundaries are not absolute. Functionally, the four levels are also distinct, again with considerable overlap. In addition, both prefrontal areas – heteromodal and supramodal – are strongly influenced by selected subcortical actions. Subcortical malfunction is a prominent source of frontal symptomatology.

Subcortical Systems with Strong Frontal Connections

'Frontal systems' disorder is a term increasingly used to denote prefrontal dysfunction without distinct pathology involving the prefrontal cortex. A subcortical locus of pathology is most often present. While many subcortical systems have strong frontal connections, their activity is not exclusively prefrontal; some subcortical structures have connections to unimodal and others (many fewer) interconnect with heteromodal association cortex. Table 4 lists six more or less well-defined subcortical systems that have powerful frontal connections. Not only can pathologic involvement of any of these systems produce behavioral changes suggesting frontal disorder but both neuropsychological testing and imaging studies in these disorders may demonstrate prefrontal dysfunction.

The clinical presentations of 'frontal systems disorders', while strongly indicating frontal dysfunction, tend to be qualitatively distinguishable from the behavioral problems produced by primary frontal pathology as outlined in table 3.

Correlation of Frontal Lobe Functions

Prefrontal functions remain difficult to demarcate. Stuss and Benson [22] suggested four major prefrontal functions – drive, sequencing, executive control and self-analysis – each acting in the supramodal manner to more basic cognitive functions. As already noted, one of these, *sequencing* (or working memory), is better considered a heteromodal function and a second, *drive,* appears strongly related to subcortical influences. Clinically derived evidence indicates that sequencing competency demands integrity of the dorsal lateral aspects of the frontal lobes, while drive is associated with midline and sagittal frontal operations. Pathology in either area produces 'frontal lobe' symptomatology but both interact so strongly in cross-modal activities that they deserve inclusion with heteromodal association cortex.

The third and fourth supramodal prefrontal functions suggested by Stuss and Benson – *executive control* and *self-analysis* – and an additional supramodal prefrontal process, *future memory*, proposed by Ingvar [24] deserve recognition as operationally distinct processes. Disturbance involving these three supramodal functions produces the most prominent symptomatology characterizing the primary frontal degenerative dementias and also appears in the behavior patterns of the secondary frontal dementias. The latter have broader manifestations, however, through strong subcortical influence on drive and sequencing as well as the supramodal operations. The symptom pictures produced by the primary and the secondary frontal degenerations, although overlapping, can be distinguished.

Discussion

Recent investigations – clinical, pathological, psychological and imaging studies – all demonstrate that a group of progressive dementing disorders have symptomatology attributable to frontal lobe malfunction. This essay proposes division of these frontal degenerative dementias into two classes: (1) primary frontal degenerative dementia follows direct impairment of prefrontal cortical tissue and produces major disturbance of highest level executive control; (2) secondary frontal degenerative dementia disrupts cortical function by impairing the strong influences of subcortical structures on frontal cortex.

References

1 American Psychiatric Association: A Psychiatric Glossary, ed 5. Washington, American Psychiatric Press, 1980.
2 Cummings JL, Benson DF: Dementia: A Clinical Approach, ed 2. Boston, Butterworth-Heinemann, 1992.
3 Kirshner HS, Tanridag O, Thurman L, Whetsell W Jr: Progressive aphasia without dementia: Two cases with focal spongiform degeneration. Ann Neurol 1987;22:527–532.
4 Mesulam MM: Slowly progressive aphasia without generalized dementia. Ann Neurol 1982;11:592–598.
5 Benson DF, Davis RJ, Snyder BD: Posterior cortical atrophy. Arch Neurol 1988;45:789–793.
6 Brun A: Frontal lobe degeneration of non-Alzheimer type. I. Neuropathology. Arch Gerontol Geriatr 1987;6:193–208.
7 Neary D, Snowden JS, Northen B, Goulding P: Dementia of frontal lobe type. J Neurol Neurosurg Psychiatry 1988;51:353–361.
8 Clark AW, White CL III, Manz HJ, Parhad IM, Curry B, Whitehouse PJ, Lehman J, Coyle JT: Primary degenerative dementia without Alzheimer pathology. Can J Neurol Sci 1986;13:462–470.
9 Dubois B, Pillon B, Legault F, Agid Y, Lhermitte F: Slowing of cognitive processing in progressive supranuclear palsy. Arch Neurol 1988;45:1194–1199.
10 Gallassi R, Montagna P, Ciardulli C, Lorusso S, Mussuto P, Stracciari A: Cognitive impairment in motor neurone disease. Acta Neurol Scand 1985;71:480–484.
11 Hudson AJ: Amyotrophic lateral sclerosis and its association with dementia, parkinsonism and other neurological disorders: A review. Brain 1981;104:217–247.
12 Jagust WJ, Reed BR, Seab JP, Kramer JH, Budinger TF: Clinical-physiologic correlates of Alzheimer's disease and frontal lobe dementia. Am J Physiol Imaging 1989;4:89–96.
13 Knopman DS, Mastri AR, Frey WH II, Sung JH, Rustan T: Dementia lacking distinctive histologic features: A common non-Alzheimer degenerative dementia. Neurology 1990;40:251–256.
14 Miller BL, Cummings JL, Villanueva-Meyer J, Boone K, Mehringer CM, Lesser IM, Mena I: Frontal lobe degeneration: Clinical, neuropsychological and SPECT characteristics. Neurology 1991;41:1374–1382.
15 Robbins TW, James M, Lange KW, Owen AM, Quinn NP, Marsden CD: Cognitive performance in multiple system atrophy. Brain 1992;115:271–291.
16 Gustafson L: Frontal lobe degeneration of non-Alzheimer type. II. Clinical picture and differential diagnosis. Arch Gerontol Geriatr 1987;6:209–223.
17 Cummings JL, Benson DF: Subcortical dementia. Arch Neurol 1984;41:874–879.
18 Baddeley A: Working memory. Science 1992;255:556–559.
19 Mesulam MM: Patterns in behavioral neuroanatomy: Association areas, the limbic system and hemispheric specialization; in Mesulam MM (ed): Principles of Behavioral Neurology. Philadelphia, Davis, 1985, pp 1–70.
20 Goldman-Rakic PS: Cellular and circuit basis of working memory in prefrontal cortex of nonhuman primates; in Uylings HBM, Van Eden CG, De Bruin JPC, Corner MA, Feenstra MGP (eds): Progress in Brain Research. Amsterdam, Elsevier, 1990, vol 85, pp 325–336.
21 Fuster JM: Temporal organization of behavior. Hum Neurobiol 1985;4:57–60.
22 Stuss DT, Benson DF: The Frontal Lobes. New York, Raven Press, 1986.
23 Fuster JM: The Prefrontal Cortex: Anatomy, Physiology and Neuropsychology of the Frontal Lobe. New York, Raven Press, 1980.
24 Ingvar DH: 'Memory of the future': An essay on the temporal organization of conscious awareness. Hum Neurobiol 1985;4:127–136.

Dementia 1993;4:154–159

D. Neary
J.S. Snowden
D.M.A. Mann

Department of Neurology, Manchester Royal Infirmary, Manchester, UK

The Clinical Pathological Correlates of Lobar Atrophy

Key Words
Dementia of frontal lobe type
Motor neurone disease
Progressive aphasia
Pick's disease
Lobar atrophy
Spongiosis
Gliosis

Abstract
Three clinical syndromes associated with fronto-temporal cerebral atrophy, studied in one centre are discussed: dementia of frontal type (DFT), DFT and motor neurone disease (MND) and progressive aphasia (PA). The pathological findings in DFT (13 brains), DFT and MND (5 brains) and PA (5 brains) permit a number of clinical pathological groupings. The nosological status of fronto-temporal atrophy is discussed with reference to the literature and it is suggested that a common underlying pathology, including Picks disease as strictly defined by the presence of inclusion bodies, underlies the clinical syndromes, each being determined by the anatomical distribution of the pathology.

Introduction

This review describes the clinical pathological correlates in three clinical syndromes arising from fronto-temporal cerebral atrophy and based on work from Manchester, UK [1–10]. These studies will address the nosological status of lobar atrophy of non-Alzheimer disease type.

The clinical syndromes reviewed reflect fronto-temporal cerebral atrophy and comprise dementia of frontal lobe type (DFT), DFT and motor neurone disease (MND), and progressive aphasia (PA). The designation DFT is used since it denotes a clinical syndrome only and does not imply any specific underlying histology.

Brain harvesting in Manchester has provided information for clinico-pathological groupings and a nosological analysis of lobar atrophy (table 1). A discussion of each of the three syndromes will include clinical descriptions with appropriate brain imaging, a delineation of the anatomical distribution of pathology within the fronto-temporal lobes and the nature of the histology.

Table 1. Patients studied

Syndrome	Patients	Family history, %	Brains
DFT	94	50	13
DFT/MND	7	14	5
PA	19	42	5

Dementia of Frontal Lobe Type

Clinical Syndrome

The syndrome appears predominantly in the presenium. In half there is a family history of a similar disorder in a first-degree relative. The presentation is of a disorder of conduct and personality and in the late stages mutism supervenes. Initially, there are few neurological signs; they comprise primitive reflexes, but with progression, striatal signs of akinesia and rigidity emerge. Survival of up to 10–15 years is not uncommon. The EEG remains

Prof. D. Neary
Department of Neurology
Manchester Royal Infirmary
Manchester, M13 9WL (UK)

1013–7424/93/0044–0154
$2.75/0

substantially normal and SPET imaging displays reduced tracer uptake in the anterior cerebral hemispheres.

Striking changes in personality and social conduct occur and individuals rapidly become incapable of managing their own affairs and lose insight into their altered condition. With progression of illness, two polarised clinical profiles emerge: an apathetic inert state contrasts with disinhibition, restlessness and inappropriate affect. Speech becomes increasingly economical, echolalic and stereotypic until mutism supervenes. Spatial and executive abilities are well preserved throughout the illness. In addition to motor perseverations of an elementary type, stereotypic and ritualistic behaviour is seen in relationship to aspects of daily living. Individuals over-eat, develop food fads and hyperoral activity. Repetitive rituals of dressing, toileting, hoarding and wandering are observed.

Anatomical Correlates and Histology

The topographical distribution of the gross histological and immunohistochemical pathologies and their severity indicate that the clinical syndrome is pathologically heterogeneous and appears to comprise three distinctive subgroups.

The first subgroup (type A) (5 brains) is characterised by a fronto-temporal atrophy defined histologically by a loss of large cortical nerve cells (chiefly from layers III and V), and a spongiform degeneration of the superficial neuropil (layer II); gliosis is minimal and restricted to subpial regions; layers III and V shows no gliosis. No distinctive changes (swellings or inclusions) within remaining nerve cells are seen. The limbic system and the striatum are affected but to a much lesser extent.

The second subgroup (type B) (5 brains) is also characterised by a fronto-temporal atrophy but which is defined by a loss of large cortical nerve cells with widespread and abundant gliosis but minimal or no spongiform change. Swollen neurones or inclusions that are both tau and ubiquitin positive are sometimes typically present in some patients, and the limbic system and striatum are more seriously damaged.

Type A and type B subgroups shared a common clinical syndrome and familial incidence.

In the third subgroup (type C) (3 brains), the brunt of the pathology is borne by the striatum with (usually) severe limbic involvement but variable cortical and nigral involvement. Immunochemistry reveals no significant changes.

The patients in type C subgroup are characterised by stereotypic and ritualistic behaviour as their predominant symptomatology and they develop striatal neurological signs early in the course of the illness. One of these 3 cases is familial.

Dementia of Frontal Lobe Type and Motor Neurone Disease

Clinical Syndrome

The patients present with typical DFT and then go on to develop the amyotrophic form of MND with widespread fasciculations, muscular weakness, wasting and bulbar palsy. The latter is responsible for death, which takes place within 3 years of onset. Neurophysiological investigations demonstrate widespread muscular denervation, the electroencephalogram remains normal and SPET imaging reveals reduced tracer in the anterior hemispheres. In the Manchester series, no patients developed extrapyramidal neurological signs.

Anatomical and Histological Changes

The structural changes are similar to type A subgroup of DFT. Atrophy is less marked and is mostly frontal with some temporal involvement characterised by a loss of large cortical nerve cells, spongiform change and mild gliosis. Limbic involvement is slight, though nigral damage is severe with heavy loss of pigmented nerve cells and intense reactive fibrous astrocytosis. No Lewy bodies are present in surviving cells. Ubiquitinated but not tau-immunoreactive inclusions are present within the frontal cortex and hippocampus (dentate gyrus). In the brain stem, the hypoglossus nucleus shows atrophy and loss of neurones. The large Betz cells of the precentral gyrus are largely preserved in number and there is no obvious demyelination within the cortico-spinal tracts. Within the anterior horn cells there is gross loss of neurones at all levels, and many of the surviving anterior horn cells contain large pale ubiquitinated inclusions within the cytoplasm. No Lewy or Pick-type inclusions are observed in any cortical or subcortical neurones.

Progressive Aphasia

Clinical Syndromes

Profile A comprises non-fluent aphasia with anomia, impaired repetition, phonemic errors with relative preservation of comprehension. In general behavioral changes akin to DFT occur late in the disease. However, the brother of one patient developed such behavioural change shortly after the onset of his linguistic presentation. Neurological signs are absent except in one patient who had progressive akinesia, rigidity and tremor of the right arm and leg. SPET images reveal reduced tracer uptake in the left cerebral hemisphere exclusively.

Profile B comprises fluent aphasia with preserved repetition, verbal paraphasias, profound problems in comprehension but with relatively preserved reading aloud and writing to dictation. A proportion of these patients go on to develop a visual associative agnosia (semantic dementia) [4]. Behavioural changes akin to DFT are sometimes observed. None have significant neurological signs. SPET images reveal bilateral reduced tracer uptake in the anterior hemispheres.

Profile C comprises patients who share affinities with both the non-fluent and fluent forms of aphasia. In these patients, behavioural change akin to DFT occur, sometimes to a marked degree. They have no neurological signs. SPET images reveal reduced tracer uptake asymmetrically in the anterior hemispheres and affecting the left side predominantly.

Anatomical and Histological Findings

In profile A patients, the brains showed markedly asymmetrical atrophy being slight and generalised on the right side but gross on the left side, particularly affecting fronto-temporal, fronto-parietal and lateral parietal/occipital regions. The left anterior temporal cortex showed 'knife edge' atrophy. The pattern of atrophy involved the hippocampus, amygdala, the caudate, putamen, globus pallidus and thalamus on the left side alone. Histologically frontal, fronto-parietal and anterior temporal cortices on the left side were severely affected and showed virtually a complete loss of large pyramidal cells from layers III and V. There was widespread spongiform change, particularly in layers II and III due to neuronal fallout. Reactive astrocytosis was mild even in severely affected regions and no Pick or Lewy type inclusion bodies were present in surviving nerve cells in any region of cortex or subcortex.

As indicated above, the brother of a patient with profile A presented with an identical linguistic breakdown but within months had developed the behavioural changes characteristic of DFT. His brain revealed asymmetrical and severe atrophy of the fronto-temporal lobes, more marked on the right than the left side. The histological changes were identical to those of his brother and the remainder of the group.

The brain of a single patient with fluent aphasia and associative agnosia (profile B) revealed a fixed brain which was grossly normal with only slight enlargement of the lateral ventricles and no obvious asymmetries of brain slices. The pathological changes were identical to those of subgroup 1 and particularly affected the middle and inferior temporal gyri with preservation of the superior temporal gyrus and parietal and occipital cortices.

The brain of one patient of profile C revealed bilateral asymmetrical atrophy chiefly affecting the left hemisphere. The temporal lobes were severely atrophied with relative sparing of the superior temporal gyrus. There was also severe involvement of the orbito-frontal cortex, whereas more anteriorly the frontal lobes were only moderately atrophied. The hippocampus was moderately atrophic and the corpus striatum, globus pallidus and thalamus grossly and bilaterally atrophied. The histological changes were compatible with those of brains of profile A and B.

Clinico-Anatomical Correlations

The clinical syndromes emerging from patients with fronto-temporal cerebral atrophy appear to reflect the topographical distribution of the pathology rather than the specific histological change, as depicted in figure 1. When the frontal lobes are bilaterally, symmetrically and predominantly affected, the syndrome of DFT emerges. When the left cerebral hemisphere is predominantly affected, the syndrome of non-fluent PA occurs. However, when the process is distributed asymmetrically, the behavioural disturbances of DFT are seen in association with linguistic disturbance, as in the patients with PA of profile C and in the more behaviourally disturbed brother with progressive non-fluent aphasia. Predominant involvement of the temporal lobes bilaterally leads to progressive fluent aphasia and associative visual agnosia. In this series of patients, MND has been associated with DFT but not with PA.

Clinico-Histological Correlations

If a distinction is made between the spongiform appearances and the gliotic change, with and without Pick bodies, then, as depicted in figure 2, the following associations can be drawn. DFT can be associated with both histologies in roughly equal proportions and with a similar familial incidence. In DFT and MND the histology is that of spongiform change. This is also the case with PA. However, the subgroup of patients with DFT who have marked stereotypic traits and early striatal neurological signs had a mixed histological picture sharing features of both types of change.

If the designation Pick's disease is used to refer to all cases of frontal temporal atrophy with both symmetrical and asymmetrical distributions of pathology, then all these clinical syndromes come within its rubric. However, if Pick's disease is more strictly defined by the histological change of astrocytic gliosis and the presence of neuronal inclusion bodies, then Pick's disease accounts for a minority of cases. Moreover the 'knife blade' appearance of circumscribed temporal atrophy does not predict the underlying histology of Pick's disease as strictly defined.

The question arises as to whether the two pathologies have an aetiological significance or whether they are simply expressions of a spectrum of pathological change, the anatomical distribution of which determines the clinical syndrome. If this is so then a number of predictions might be advanced.

(1) Cases of progressive aphasia ought to occur in association with the histology of Pick's disease as strictly described (gliosis, inclusion bodies and swollen cells).

(2) An asymmetrical distribution of the spongiform pathology in cases with MND might be expected to be associated with the syndrome of progressive aphasia.

(3) Some cases with DFT/MND ought to have the histology of Pick's disease.

(4) If genetic factors underlie the spectrum of histologies then familial cases of each syndrome and histology ought to occur. The literature will be reviewed in order to address these issues.

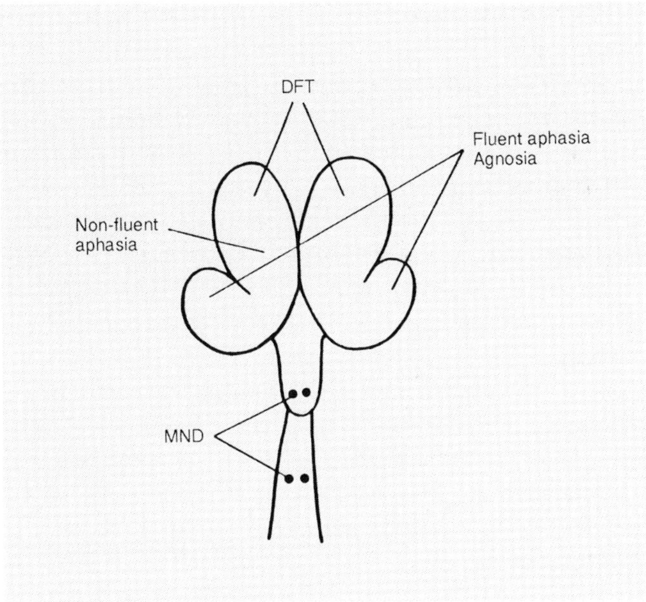

1

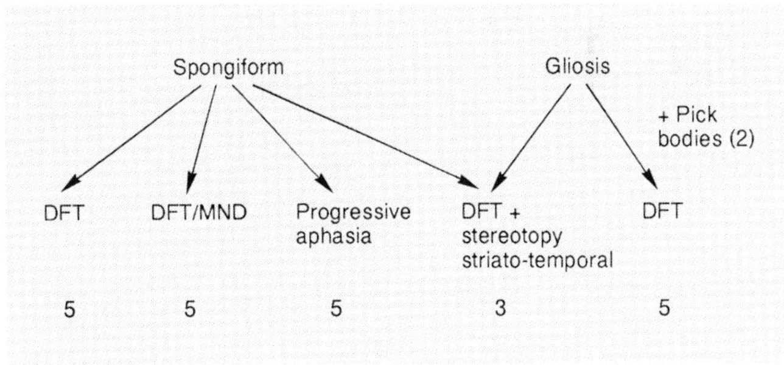

2

Fig. 1. Clinical-anatomical relationships.
Fig. 2. Clinical-histological relationships in labor atrophy.

Review of the Literature

Dementia of Frontal Lobe Type

Gustafson [11], Brun [12] and Risberg [13] described 20 cases from Lund. They have used the term 'frontal lobe degeneration' (FLD) to refer to the underlying histology of neuronal cell loss and spongiform appearances, in the absence of 'inflated cells and inclusions'. The latter are held to define Pick's disease. There were 'only small and non systematic clinical differences between ... FLD and Pick's cases'. Thus the same clinical syndrome shares two seemingly distinct pathologies.

Tissot et al. [14] in reviewing Pick's disease describe a clinical syndrome consonant with DFT. They described three categories of histological change: gliosis, gliosis with neuronal swellings (NS) and gliosis with NS and argyrophilic inclusions (AI). They assigned an overactive disinhibited group of patients to a corresponding pathology chiefly in the orbital frontal and temporal lobes. By contrast inert, apathetic patients with extrapyramidal signs had predominant pathology in the dorso-frontal cortex and basal ganglia. Neurological extrapyramidal signs were not described in the Lund patients. However, prolonged follow-up in Manchester has indicated that the majority of patients eventually develop akinesia and rigidity, in keeping with the underlying striatal involvement. Moreover, in 3 patients with early striatal change and stereotypic behaviour, the striatum and limbic-temporal lobe were chiefly affected. Such patients which represent a subgroup of DFT, would presumably be excluded from FLD as pathologically defined. In both Lund and Manchester there was a high familial incidence, as in 'familial dementia of adult onset' described by Kim et al. [15] in 4 of 10 siblings of an Italian family.

Dementia of Frontal Lobe Type/Motor Neurone Disease

There are few detailed neuropsychological studies of patients with dementia and MND or ALS. However, Gustafson [11] noted that one FLD patient 'showed evidence of motor neurone disease'. Mitsuyama [16] described 'presenile dementia with motor neurone disease in Japan'. In reviewing the extensive Japanese literature, Morita et al. [17] write 'dementia ... is the frontal temporal type, or "anterior dementia". Morita et al. recorded extrapyramidal signs in 27% of patients. Since the substantia nigra is characteristically degenerate in DFT/MND, the emergence of parkinsonian signs might be anticipated to occur earlier in DFT/MND.

However, the development of bulbar palsy is likely to dictate the early death of patients who may have insufficient time to manifest extrapyramidal signs. This is supported by the occurrence of the latter in cases of longer duration [17]. Moreover of patients with striatal signs 88% had significant degeneration of the substantia nigra. This subgroup of patients with extrapyramidal signs is commented on by Salazar et al. [18] in their studies of the syndromes 'ALS and dementia'.

It is puzzling that the fronto-temporal atrophy with spongiform appearances is so common a finding in this syndrome. Knopman et al. [20] in assessing forms of non-Alzheimer's disease dementia from a brain bank referred to 'dementia lacking distinctive histological features (DLDH)' to describe the non-specific large neuronal cell loss and spongiform appearances. Three fifths of patients with DLDH pathology also had that of MND. Again there was a familial incidence, half the cases having a family history of dementia, and one a family history of MND. In the Manchester series, one patient with DFT/MND had a mother with dementia, but not MND. The importance of genetic factors is again highlighted in this syndrome by Constantinidis' [21] report of 4 members of 2 generations who developed characteristic DFT and later MND. In 2 autopsied cases, there was predominant fronto-temporal atrophy, asymmetrically favouring the left hemisphere. The histological findings were not of spongiosis, but of gliosis, neuronal cell loss and ballooned neurones, in the absence of inclusion bodies. Brion et al. [22] have also noted sporadic cases of DFT/MND with gliotic rather than spongiform histology. Thus the latter in DFT/MND is not an invariable finding.

Progressive Aphasia

Case descriptions have proliferated but there have been few clinico-pathological studies. Pick's original clinical description of a case of lobar atrophy [23] was of progressive linguistic impairment. Interestingly, the first modern case of 'pre-senile dementia presenting as aphasia', described by Wechsler [24], subsequently came to autopsy [25] and proved to have fronto-temporal atrophy, principally left sided with a histology of Pick's disease as strictly defined. A subsequent case with very similar clinical and pathological findings has been described [26].

The familial nature of progressive aphasia has been attested to by Morris et al. [28] who use the term 'hereditary dysphasic dementia'. The majority of cases of PA display, histologically, the spongiform appearances rather than Pick's disease and in one of two cases [29] there was also wasting and fasciculations of the upper and lower limbs as well as a similar disease in the patient's mother. Thus the link between PA and MND is further established.

Conclusion

In general the literature supports the formulation that the distinctive clinical syndromes of lobar atrophy are dictated by anatomy and that the syndromes do not necessarily predict the precise histology. The latter appears to represent a spectrum of pathological change, rather than demarcated entities, especially since familial cases exist for each syndrome and for each histological type.

It is clear from the foregoing that clinical terms cannot be used interchangeably with pathological designations. DFT, DFT/MND and PA refer to clinical syndromes whereas FLD, DLDH and PD denote particular histologies. There is, as yet, no accepted definition of the pathological criteria for Pick's disease. It was Alzheimer [30] not Pick who referred to 'ballooned cells', 'argentophilic globes' and 'spongi cortico wasting'. Some authors simply accept circumscribed fronto-temporal atrophy without characteristic histology [31, 32]. Others stipulate the presence of ballooning of neurones in addition to the macroscopic change [33]. More recently it has been proposed [15, 34] that a combination of progressive dementia, lobar atrophy and neuronal argentophilic inclusion (Pick) bodies be diagnostic of Pick's disease. Since fronto-temporal degeneration is heterogenous and can occur in a minority of cases of Alzheimer disease and Creutzfeldt-Jakob disease [12], and since ballooned neurones occur in a variety of neurodegenerative conditions [35, 36], it might be suggested that the presence of Pick inclusion bodies represents the conclusive histology since they are rarely found in other conditions [37].

If descriptive distinctions are made between clinical syndromes, anatomical distributions of atrophy and histological changes, then Pick's disease can be viewed as a specific histology which can underlie fronto-temporal atrophy in the syndromes of DFT, DFT/MND and PA. Other histologies such as FLD and DLDH are likely to reflect stages in, rather than departures from a common pathological process. Prefixing eponyms or acronyms to the pathology is not explanatory. The processes leading to spongiosis and gliosis require delineation and it remains to be explained whether neuronal inclusion bodies vanish from tissues along with neuronal cell loss and astrocytosis.

The tasks for the future are to determine the nature of the differing pathological changes underlying lobar atrophy and, given the high familial incidence, to search for a molecular biological basis which might explain them.

References

1 Neary D, Snowden JS, Bowen DM, et al: Neuropsychological syndromes in presenile dementia due to cerebral atrophy. J Neurol Neurosurg Psychiatry 1986;49:163–174.
2 Neary D, Snowden JS, Shields RA, et al: Single photon emission tomography using ^{99m}Tc-HM-PAO in the investigation of dementia. J Neurol Neurosurg Psychiatry 1987;50:1101–1109.
3 Neary D, Snowden JS, Northen B, Goulding PJ: Dementia of frontal lobe type. J Neurol Neurosurg Psychiatry 1988;51:353–361.
4 Snowden JS, Goulding PJ, Neary D: Semantic dementia: A form of circumscribed cerebral atrophy. Behav Neurol 1989;2:167–182.
5 Goulding PJ, Northen B, Snowden JS, et al: Progressive aphasia with right-sided extrapyramidal signs: Another manifestation of localised cerebral atrophy. J Neurol Neurosurg Psychiatry 1989;52:128–130.
6 Northen B, Hopcutt B, Griffiths H: Progressive aphasia without generalised dementia. Aphasiology 1990;4:55–65.
7 Neary D, Snowden JS, Mann DMA, et al: Frontal lobe dementia and motor neuron disease. J Neurol Neurosurg Psychiatry 1990;53: 23–32.
8 Neary D: Non-Alzheimer's disease forms of cerebral atrophy. J Neurol Neurosurg Psychiatry 1990;53:929–931.
9 Snowden JS, Neary D, Mann DMA, et al: Progressive language disorder due to lobar atrophy. Ann Neurol 1992;31:174–183.
10 Mann DMA, South PW, Snowden JS, Neary D: Dementia of frontal lobe type: Neuropathology and immunohistochemistry. J Neurol Neurosurg Psychiatry, in press.
11 Gustafson L: Frontal lobe degeneration of non-Alzheimer type. II. Clinical picture and differential diagnosis. Arch Gerontol Geriatr 1987;6: 193–208.
12 Brun A: Frontal lobe degeneration of non-Alzheimer's type: Neuropathology. Arch Gerontol Geriatr 1987;6:193–208.
13 Risberg J: Frontal lobe degeneration of non-Alzheimer type. III. Regional cerebral blood flow. Arch Gerontol Geriatr 1987;6:225–233.
14 Tissot R, Constantinidis J, Richard J, Frederiks JAM (ed): Pick's Disease. Handbook of Clinical Neurology. Amsterdam, Elsevier Science Publishers, 1985, vol 2 (46), Chapt 132, pp 233–246.
15 Kim RC, Collins GH, Paris JE: Familial dementia of adult onset with pathological findings on a 'non-specific' nature. Brain 1981;104: 61–78.
16 Mitsuyama Y: Presenile dementia with motor neuron disease in Japan: Clinico-pathological review of 26 cases. J Neurol Neurosurg Psychiatry 1984;47:953–959.
17 Morita K, Kaiya H, Ikeda T, Namba M: Presenile dementia combined with amyotrophy: A review of 34 Japanese cases. Arch Gerontol Geriatr 1987;6:263–277.
18 Salazar AM, Masters CL, Gajdusek C, Gibbs CJ: Syndromes of ALS and dementia: Relation to Creutzfeldt-Jakob disease. Ann Neurol 1983;14:17–26.
19 Allen IV, Dermott E, Connolly JH, Hurwitz LJ: A study of a patient with the amyotrophic form of Creutzfeldt-Jakob disease. Brain 1971;94: 715–724.
20 Knopman DA, Mastri AR, Frey WH, et al: Dementia lacking distinctive histological features: A common non-Alzheimer degenerative dementia. Neurology 1990;40:251–256.
21 Constantinidis J: Syndrome familial: association de maladie de Pick et sclérose latérale amyotrophique. Encéphale 1987;13:285–293.
22 Brion S, Psimaras A, Chevalier JF, et al: L'association maladie de Pick et sclérose latérale amyotrophique. Etude d'un cas anatomo-clinique et revue de la littérature. Encéphale 1980; 6:250–286.
23 Pick A: Über die Beziehungen der senilen Hirnatrophie zur Aphasie. Prager Med Wochenschr 1892;17:165–167.
24 Wechsler AF: Presenile dementia presenting as aphasia. J Neurol Neurosurg Psychiatry 1977; 40:303–305.
25 Wechsler AF, Verity MA: Pick's disease. A clinical computed tomographic and histological study with Golgi impregnation observations. Arch Neurol 1982;39:287–290.
26 Graff-Radford NR, Damasio AR, Damasio H, et al: Progressive aphasia in a patient with Pick's disease. Neurology 1990;40:620–626.
27 Mesulam MM: Slowly progressive aphasia without generalised dementia. Ann Neurol 1982;11:592–598.
28 Morris JC, Munroe C, Barker BQ, Wright D: Hereditary dysphasic dementia and the Pick-Alzheimer spectrum. Ann Neurol 1984;16: 455–466.
29 Kirshner H, Ogurz T, Lawrence T, Whetsell WO: Progressive aphasia without dementia. Two cases with focal spongiform degeneration. Ann Neurol 1987;22:527–532.
30 Alzheimer A: Über eigenartige Krankheitsfälle des späteren Alters. Z Gesamte Neurol Psychiatr 1911;4:356–385.
31 Malamud N, Boyd DA: Pick's disease with atrophy of the temporal lobes: A clinicopathological study. Arch Neurol Psychiatry 1940;43: 210–222.
32 Constantinidis J, Richard J, Tissot R: Pick's disease: Histological and clinical correlations. Eur Neurol 1987;11:208–217.
33 Lindgren AKH: The patho-anatomical classification of morbus Alzheimer and morbus Pick. Acta Psychiatr Neurol Scand 1952;suppl 81: 118–152.
34 Verity MA, Wechsler AF: Progressive subcortical gliosis of Neumann: A clinicopathological study of 2 cases with review. Arch Gerontol Geriatr 1987;6:245–261.
35 Lowe J, Errington DR, Lennox G, et al: Ballooned neurons in several neurodegenerative diseases and stroke contain d crystallin. Neuropathol Appl Neurobiol 1992;18:341–350.
36 Kato S, Hirani A, Umahara T, et al: Comparative immunohistochemical study on the expression of crystallin ubiquitin and stress-response protein 27 in ballooned neurons in various disorders. Neuropathol Appl Neurobiol 1992;18:335–340.
37 Clark AW, Manz HJ, White C, et al: Cortical degeneration with swollen chromatolytic neurons: Its relationship to Pick's disease. J Neuropathol Exp Neurol 1986;45:268–284.
38 Green J, Morris JC, Sandson J, et al: Progressive aphasia: A precursor of global dementia. Neurology 1990;40:423–429.

Dementia 1993;4:160–162

Ulla Passant
Lars Gustafson
Arne Brun

Department of Psychogeriatrics and Pathology, University Hospital, Lund, Sweden

Spectrum of Frontal Lobe Dementia in a Swedish Family

Key Words
Frontal lobe dementia of non-Alzheimer type (FLD)
Family study
Heredity
Neuropathological findings
Clinical characteristics

Abstract
The etiology of frontal lobe dementia of non-Alzheimer type (FLD) is still unknown. There is strong evidence of genetic factors with positive heredity. In this paper, a Swedish family, with several generations affected by FLD is described. In 3 patients typical FLD was confirmed postmortem. The clinical and neuropathological similarities between the patients are impressive.

Introduction

The etiology of frontal lobe dementia of non-Alzheimer type (FLD) is still unknown. There is however strong evidence of genetic factors with positive heredity for dementia reported in about 50% [1–3]. As an illustration of heredity in FLD, we present a pedigree of a Swedish family with several generations affected by dementia (fig. 1).

The diagnosis was based on the patient's history, neuropsychiatric and neuropsychological findings. In the last generation, the diagnosis was supported by brain-imaging techniques, CT, rCBF, SPECT and EEG. In 3 patients, typical FLD was confirmed postmortem. The clinical and neuropathological similarities between the patients were striking.

The early stage was dominated by change and deterioration of personality and behaviour, lack of concern and disinhibition. Later on, there were changes in speech with stereotyped phrases and often echolalia. Motor disturbances were not prominent, but in the final stage before death, the patients very often became bedridden, with mutism and amimia. In at least one of the cases, death was caused by hyperphagia and aspiration.

The neuropathological findings were similar in the 3 cases and representative of FLD, as defined originally [4, 5]: Macroscopically, there was a slight frontal lobe atrophy with frontal ventricular widening. Microscopic examination showed nerve cell loss and a slight gliosis in superficial portions of the frontal cortex. There were no Pick bodies or Alzheimer plaques or tangles beyond what is physiological for age and no Lewy bodies were found. White matter changes consisted of a mild astrocytic gliosis. The striatum showed mild and questionable changes. In the brain stem the substantia nigra showed a mild to moderate loss of neurons. The cerebellum was unremarkable for age.

Subjects and Methods

In this family 10 affected members (8 women and 2 men) have so far been identified. Two members are still living. The average age of onset (n = 8) was 53 years (range 43–65 years), the average age at death (n = 8) was 68 years (range 55–88 years) and duration of illness (n = 7) was 12 years (range 5–21 years) (table 1).

Ulla Passant
Department of Psychogeriatrics
University Hospital
Box 638
S-220 09 Lund (Sweden)

1013–7424/93/0044–0160
$2.75/0

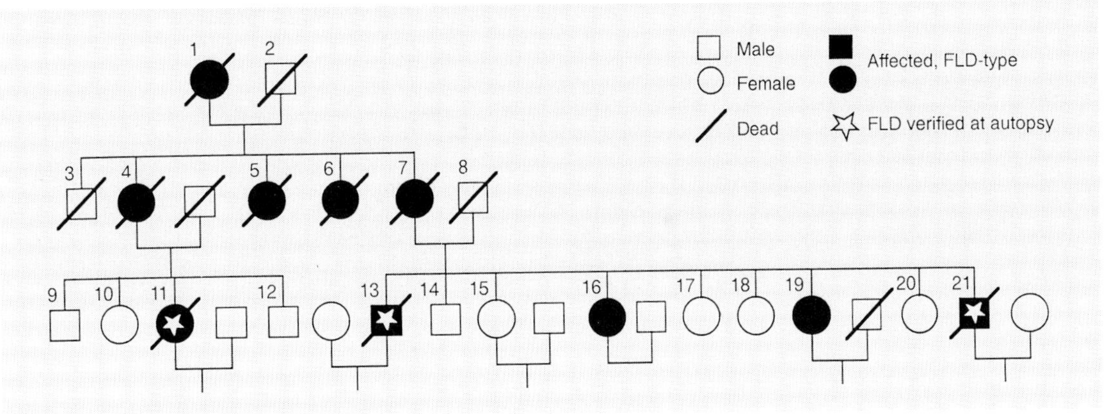

Fig. 1. Pedigree of a family with FLD.

Case Reports

Case 1. This woman was born 1858, and had been demented for many years according to her children and other relatives. She suffered a stroke during the last year of her life and died at the age of 88.

Case 2. The husband of case 1, born 1861, died at the age of 49 years from a cardiac disease.

Case 4. At the age of 57, a change was noted in the personality and behaviour of this woman. She became very restless, neglectful, disinhibited and socially embarrassing. She spent a lot of time visiting unknown people, laughing, chatting, telling jokes and confabulating. 2 years later, she could not be taken care of at home any longer. Her expressive speech became reduced and she used only a limited number of phrases. She showed verbal as well as physical aggressiveness. Five years after onset, she was still fully orientated. Later on, she became mutistic. The EEG at this time was normal. The disease left her bedridden for several years. She died at 69 years of age.

Case 5. According to her relatives, this woman had a 10-year history of dementia before her death at the age of 70. The clinical picture was similar to that of case number 7.

Case 6. This woman lived extremely isolated in a small cottage in the forest. She did not have much contact with people. It was reported that her personality changed markedly at the age of 65. She became restless, irritable and sometimes aggressive. She showed a stereotyped behaviour. She managed to live in her cottage for many years. Her spatial abilities were intact and physically she was in good condition. During the last year before her death, at the age of 86, she had a stroke.

Case 7. At the age of 55, this woman presented progressive deterioration of her personality with neglect of personal hygiene, family and household. Her mood changed rapidly and she became very quarrelsome and aggressive. She had periods of apathy and depression with suicidal thoughts. She also had auditory hallucinations. Already after 1 year she was referred to a mental hospital. Her speech had changed with increased verbal productivity, but she only produced a limited number of phrases which she was also singing. Later on, she developed fragmented echolalia. She showed no insight. Her ability to find her way around the ward and hospital was normal. Her oral behaviour changed and she ate almost everything she could find. One year before death she became bedridden and required total nursing care. She died at the age of 61 years.

Table 1. Characteristics of probands

Pedigree No.	Sex	Age of onset	Age at death	Duration of illness
1	F	?	88	?
4	F	57	69	12
5	F	60	70	10
6	F	65	86	21
7	F	55	61	6
11	F	50	55	5
13	M	46	61	15
16	F	?	living (73)	–
19	F	52	living (65)	–
21	M	43	60	17

Case 11. This woman's husband reported a change in her personality when she was 50. She became unconcerned about herself, her family and things that had interested her earlier. She also reported visual hallucinations and started to confabulate. Her speech changed rapidly to stereotyped phrases. Her memory and spatial functions were normal. Later she became aggressive. She did not show any insight at all and was very unconcerned about everything. She also had periods of apathy. She spent most of the last 2 years of her life in hospital. Her speech was dominated by perseverations and echolalia. Her oral behaviour changed and she choked to death due to aspiration of large pieces of food. She was then 55 years old.

The EEG at the age of 53 was normal. One year later, mild abnormalities were seen. rCBF at the age of 53 showed frontal pathology. CT scan at the age of 55 showed cortical atrophy with frontal accentuation. Autopsy confirmed the diagnosis FLD.

Case 13. At the age of 46 this man had several depressive episodes with suicidal thoughts. He also became suspicious about most things, whether it concerned job or family. He also started to neglect his family. A few years later, disinhibition and compulsive behaviour were noticed. He was involved in several severe traffic accidents and showed overactive and altered sexual behaviour. He also started to drink alcohol quite heavily, which was new. No memory impairment was reported and spatial functions were normal. Later, his speech as well as his behaviour became very stereotyped. He spoke only about 10 phrases, which he kept repeating all day. His oral behaviour changed, and he put everything which he could find in his mouth. One year before his death, he was more or less mute. In contrast to most other affected members, he was physically mobile and walking around until he died at the age of 61 years.

EEG recordings were repeatedly normal until he was 60. Pneumoencephalography at the age of 57 showed slight cortical atrophy. Neuropathology confirmed the diagnosis FLD.

Case 16. According to her relatives, this woman has been demented for several years. She is now 73 years old (1992). The information about her clinical picture is limited. She has had no medical contact so far and has been looked after by her husband.

Case 19. At the age of 52, this woman suddenly started to neglect her job, family and other social contacts. She became very restless. Her speech changed quite early to stereotyped phrases. Due to lack of insight she ran into several unpleasant incidents at work. Her orientation was preserved and no memory impairment was reported. Later, her conversation was dominated by echolalia. Her oral behaviour changed and she put everything in her mouth and ate greedily. Her movements became very stereotyped. She has been mute for 5 years, is now bedridden and requires total nursing care. She is now 65 years old (1992).

Her EEG 1 year after onset was normal. Five years after onset, it showed mild abnormalities. CT at the age of 53 showed slight central atrophy. rCBF at the age of 54 showed frontal pathology. Subsequent repeated rCBF measurements showed progress of the frontal pathology. SPECT at the age of 63 showed severe frontal pathology.

Case 21. Clinical symptoms were noticed in this male at the age of 43. His family noticed personality changes with restlessness, explosive temper over slightest things and increased alcohol consumption. He had no insight into his changed behaviour. His lack of insight and disinhibition led to shoplifting and impulsive economic transactions which also led to tragic consequences for the family.

He also had tactile and visual hallucinations with social consequences. Orientation in time and space was normal and no memory impairment was noticed. He was very restless, and walked long distances without goals, but always finding his way. His speech consisted of stereotyped phrases and echolalia. One year before death hardly any speech was left and he was amimic. He required total nursing care, and died at the age of 60.

EEG 1 year before death was pathological. CT, rCBF/SPECT at the age of 58 showed frontal pathology. Neuropathology confirmed the diagnosis FLD.

Results

A positive heredity for FLD was found in this family, with 10 affected members in three generations. The clinical picture, although limited in some cases, is strikingly similar and in agreement with earlier studies of FLD [1–3]. The clinical characteristics, such as age of onset, age at death and duration of illness are also in accordance with previous studies [1, 2].

Moreover, brain imaging available in several cases, showed frontal pathology with relatively preserved postcentral areas. The neuropathology in 3 cases of the third generation confirmed the FLD diagnosis.

Comments

FLD is to our experience the second most common primary degenerative dementia with a characteristic clinical picture and a consistent pathology.

The aim of our presentation has been to draw attention to heredity as one important etiological factor. Other studies of FLD have reported positive heredity in about 50% of first-degree relatives [1, 2]. Further research on this family will focus on identification of new cares and continuous follow-up on affected members.

Acknowledgements

The present study was supported by the Swedish Medical Research Council (grant 3950).

We are grateful to Siv Karlsson for the illustrations and to Anette Welin for secretarial help.

References

1 Gustafson L: Frontal lobe degeneration of non-Alzheimer type. II. Clinical picture and differential diagnosis. Arch Gerontol Geriatr 1987;6: 209–223.
2 Neary D: Dementia of frontal type. J Am Geriatr Soc 1990;38:71–72.
3 Knopman DS, Mastri AR, Frey WH, et al: Dementia lacking distinctive histologic features: A common non-Alzheimer degenerative dementia. Neurology 1990;40:251–256.
4 Brun A: Frontal lobe degeneration of non-Alzheimer type. I. Neuropathology. Arch Gerontol Geriatr 1987;6:193–208.
5 Brun A: Dementia of frontal lobe type; in Racagni et al (eds): Biological Psychiatry. Amsterdam, Elsevier, 1991, vol 2, 127–128.
6 Neary D, Snowden JS, Northen B, Gouldin P: Dementia of frontal lope type. Neurol Neurosurg Psychiat 1988;51:353–361.

Dementia 1993;4:163–166

Exclusion Mapping in Familial Non-Specific Dementia

Jeremy Brown [a, d]
Susanne Gydesen [b]
Sven Asger Sorensen [b]
Arne Brun [c]
Karen Duff [a]
Henry Houlden [a]
Liana Fidani [a]
Sunita Kullkarni [a]
Juris Cummings [a]
Alison Goate [a]
Martin Rossor [d]
John Hardy [a]

[a] Department of Biochemistry and Molecular Genetics, St. Mary's Hospital Medical School, London, UK;
[b] Institute of Medical Genetics, Panum Institute, University of Copenhagen, Denmark;
[c] Department of Neuropathology, University Hospital, Lund, Sweden;
[d] Department of Neurology, St. Mary's Hospital, London, UK

Key Words
Frontal lobe dementia
Non-specific dementia
Pick's disease
Microsatellite sequences
Linkage analysis

Abstract
We present genetic linkage data in a large family in which non-specific dementia is inherited as an autosomal dominant trait. We have analyzed 45 highly polymorphic microsatellite sequences and excluded a quarter of the genome as the site of the pathogenic mutation in this family.

Introduction

Recently, several groups have described patients with dementia who at autopsy lack specific neuropathological features [1–5]. The majority of these 'non-specific' dementias have clinical and pathological evidence of frontal lobe dysfunction. Different authors have used various names for this group of patients; the most widely used is frontal lobe dementia of the non-Alzheimer type (FLD). Many patients have a positive family history [3, 6] and one large pedigree has been described in which the disease gene segregates in an autosomal dominant fashion with high penetrance [4]. We present molecular genetic findings in this family.

Familial non-specific dementias may be a heterogeneous group of disorders rather than a single disease so we have concentrated work on this one pedigree. We have already excluded the two genes known to carry mutations which can cause dementia [Brown et al., unpubl. data]: the amyloid precursor protein (APP) gene and the prion protein gene and three candidate regions for 'dementia genes': the proximal short arm of chromosome 21 (early-onset Alzheimer's disease [7]), the short arm of chromosome 4 (Huntington's disease [8]) and the proximal long arm of chromosome 19 (late-onset Alzheimer's disease [9]). We have now started a genome search for a linked marker using highly polymorphic microsatellite repeat sequences as probes. We report on results with the first 45 of these probes. We have analyzed microsatellite sequences on 21 of the 22 autosomes and excluded one quarter of the genome as the possible site of the disease gene.

Materials and Methods

Clinico-pathological details of this family have been published previously [4]. Affected individuals have clinical features suggestive of frontal lobe disease. Post mortem examination in four individuals showed generalized cerebral atrophy affecting the frontal lobes severely without specific pathological changes. The pedigree is

Jeremy Brown
Department of Biochemistry and Molecular Genetics
St. Mary's Hospital Medical School
Norfolk Place
London W2 1PG (UK)

1013–7424/93/0044–0163
$2.75/0

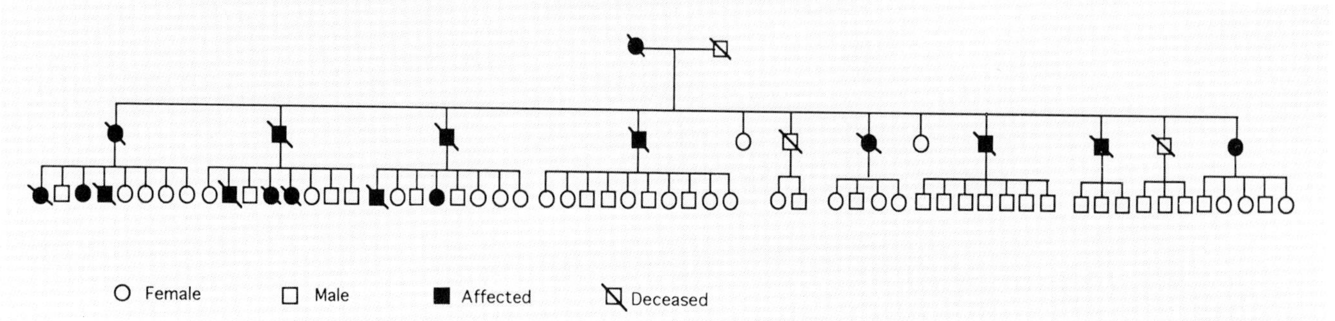

Fig. 1. Pedigree of a large family with NSD. Only three generations are shown for clarity.

shown in figure 1. 17 patients have been affected in the family in 3 generations, over 100 individuals are at risk. We have obtained blood samples from 42 individuals, 6 of them affected.

Molecular Genetics

DNA was extracted from whole blood or lymphoblasts. Highly polymorphic microsatellite sequences were amplified by the polymerase chain reaction (PCR) using specific primers whose sequence was obtained from published sources (table 1). PCR conditions were either as published with the primer sequences or as described by Weber and May [10]. ^{35}S was included in the reaction mix to label the product. The product was run on 6% denaturing polyacrylamide gel and the resultant bands sized by autoradiography using M13 phage sequence.

Linkage Analysis

The computer program LINKAGE was used for the linkage analysis, the subprogram MLINK was used for two-point analyses and the subprogram LINKMAP for multipoint analyses. Evidence against linkage was expressed as a lod score. A lod score of less than −2 represents a significant probability that there is no linkage. Allele frequencies were obtained from published sources (table 1). Equal recombination fractions were used for both sexes. Seven liability classes were calculated from the age-incidence curve in the pedigree. The phenocopy rate was estimated at 1 in 10,000. The penetrance was set at 99% by 70 years of age. The distance excluded was calculated from the recombination fraction using Haldane's mapping function.

Results

Results of two-point analyses are shown in figure 1. The total exclusion to −2 with these 45 probes and 6 dinucleotide repeats on chromosomes 19, 20 and 21 [Brown et al., unpubl. data] is approximately 700 cM. The average exclusion per probe is 14 cM (7 cM in each direction).

Discussion

We have not found linkage in this family but have excluded one quarter of the genome as the site of the causative mutation for non-specific dementia. The average exclusion of 14 cM per probe suggests that about 200 microsatellite sequences will be needed to cover the whole genome. Multipoint analyses between adjacent probes may reduce this number.

The maximum lod score obtained is +1 for the tetranucleotide repeat in the adenosine deaminase (ADA) gene on chromosome 20. We analyzed probes which map adjacent to this locus (D20S17 and cystatin) and used multipoint linkage analysis to exclude this region. A similar approach excluded the distal long arm of chromosome 14 where two adjacent probes yield small positive lod scores.

Our approach should lead to the identification of a linked genetic marker in this family. This will allow screening of families with similar phenotypes – FLD, atypical Pick's disease and non-specific dementias to ascertain whether they are caused by mutations in the same region. This will start a classification of familial frontal lobe/non-specific dementias based on their genetic aetiology and permit exploration of their relationship to typical and atypical familial forms of Pick's disease.

Acknowledgments

J. B. was supported by the Medical Research Council and Action Research. S. G. was supported by the Foundation of Else and Svend Madsen, Denmark.

Table 1. Exclusion mapping

Probe	Position	Lod score				Exclusion cM
		θ = 0	θ = 0.05	θ = 0.10	θ = 0.15	
D1S104	1q21–q23	−11.3	−3.9	−2.4	−1.6	15 [11]
D1S103	1q32–q44	−11.3	−3.5	−2.2	−1.4	13 [12]
D2S72	2	−5.1	−1.2	−0.7	−0.4	2 [13]
GCG	2q36–q37	−6.4	−1.0	−0.3	0.0	2 [14]
D3S11	3p21	−9.2	−3.0	−1.7	−1.0	8 [15]
D3S196	3q27–q28	−9.6	−1.9	−0.7	−0.2	4 [16]
HOX7	4p16.3–p16.1	−4.9	−0.7	−0.3	−0.1	2 [17]
D4S174	4p15–p11	−10.6	−3.7	−2.1	−1.2	11 [18]
D4S171	4q33–35	−16.4	−5.1	−3.1	−2.0	18 [19]
D5S208	5p15.3–p15.1	−8.1	−2.0	−1.2	−0.8	5 [20]
D5S107	5q11.2–q13.3	−8.2	−1.8	−0.9	−0.4	4 [21]
D5S39	5q11.2–q13.3	−1.4	−0.3	0.0	+0.1	0 [22]
D5S210	5q31.3–q33.3	−5.6	−1.1	−0.8	−0.5	1 [23]
FX111A	6p25–p24	−3.2	−0.5	−0.0	+0.3	0 [25]
D6S89	6p24–p23	−15.8	−3.0	−1.7	−1.0	8 [24]
HTF11D	6	−12.7	−4.2	−2.6	−1.7	15 [26]
D7S440	7	−2.4	+0.1	+0.3	+0.4	0 [27]
PENK	8q23–q24	−0.5	−0.5	−0.4	−0.4	0 [29]
D8S87	8p12	+0.4	+0.3	+0.3	+0.2	0 [28]
D8S85	8q21–q22	−17.2	−4.7	−2.9	−1.9	16 [28]
D9S55	9p12	−10.2	−3.8	−2.5	−1.7	15 [30]
ASS	9q34.1	−16.1	−4.9	−3.0	−2.0	18 [31]
D10S89	10pter–p11.2	+0.1	+0.1	+0.1	0.0	0 [32]
D10S169	10q11.2–qter	−0.4	−0.3	−0.2	−0.2	0 [32]
TH	11p15.5	−14.7	−4.1	−2.4	−1.5	14 [33]
D11S527	11q13.5	−11.0	−2.7	−1.5	−0.9	8 [34]
CD3D	11q23	−15.8	−4.4	−2.7	−1.8	15 [35]
VWF	12pter–p12	−5.7	−2.0	−1.3	−0.9	5 [36]
D13S71	13	−10.1	−2.2	−1.3	−0.9	6 [37]
D14S34	14	−1.3	−0.1	+0.3	+0.4	0 [38]
D14S48	14q	−0.4	−0.1	0.0	0.0	0 [39]
D14S49	14q	−6.4	−1.8	−1.0	−0.5	4 [39]
D14S53	14q	−12.6	−2.9	−1.5	−0.8	8 [39]
D14S54	14q	−6.7	−2.5	−1.5	−1.0	8 [39]
D14S51	14q32	−13.6	−3.3	−2.0	−1.3	11 [39]
FES	15q25–qter	−3.8	−1.2	−0.8	−0.6	0 [40]
D16S261	16q	−9.2	−2.6	−1.6	−1.1	8 [41]
D16S265	16q	−13.3	−3.4	−2.0	−1.3	11 [41]
D17S250	17q11.2–q12	−9.2	−3.3	−2.0	−1.3	11 [42]
D20S17	20q12–q13.1	−10.5	−1.8	−0.9	−0.4	4 [43]
ADA	20q12–q13.11	−1.9	+0.7	+1.0	+1.0	0 [44]
CSTP	20q13.3	−12.9	−3.7	−2.2	−1.4	13 [45]
CYST	20q13.3	−13.5	−3.3	−1.9	−1.1	10 [46]
CYP2D	22q11.2–qter	−14.3	−1.5	−0.5	−0.1	4 [47]
D22S156	22q	−9.2	−2.8	−1.8	−1.2	9 [48]

References

1 Kim RC, Collins GH, Parisi JE, Wright AW, Chu YB: Familial dementia of adult onset with pathological findings of a 'nonspecific' nature. Brain 1981;104:61–78
2 Brun A: Frontal lobe degeneration of non-Alzheimer type. I. Neuropathology. Arch Gerontol Geriatr 1987;6:193–207.
3 Gustafson L: Frontal lobe degeneration of non-Alzheimer type. II. Clinical picture and differential diagnosis. Arch Gerontol Geriatr 1987;6: 209–233.
4 Gydesen S, Hagen S, Klinken L, Abelskov J, Sorenson SA: Neuropsychiatric studies in a family with presenile dementia different from Alzheimer and Pick disease. Acta Psychiatr Scand 1987;76:276–284.
5 Neary D, Snowden JS, Northen B, Goulding P: Dementia of the frontal lobe type. J Neurol Neurosurg Psychiatry 1988;51:353–361.
6 Neary D: Non-Alzheimer's disease forms of cerebral atrophy. J Neurol Neurosurg Psychiatry 1990;53:929–931.
7 St George Hyslop P and 63 others. Genetic linkage studies suggest that Alzheimer's disease is not a single homogeneous disorder. Nature 1990;347:194–197.
8 Wasmuth JJ, Hewitt J, Smith B, Allard D, Haines JL, Skarecky D, Partlow E, Hayden MR: A highly polymorphic locus very tightly linked to the Huntington's disease gene. Nature 1988;332:734–736.
9 Pericak-Vance MA, Bebout JL, Gaskell PC, Yamaoka LH, Hung W-Y, Alberts MJ, Walker AP, Bartlett RJ, Haynes CA, Welsh KA, Earl NL, Heyman A, Clark CM, Roses AD: Linkage studies in familial Alzheimer disease: Evidence for chromosome 19 linkage. Am J Hum Genet 1991;48:1034–1050.
10 Weber JL, May PE: Abundant class of human DNA polymorphisms which can be typed using the polymerase chain reaction. Am J Hum Genet 1989;44:388–396.
11 Weber JL, Kwitek AE, May PE: Dinucleotide repeat polymorphism at the D1S104 locus. Nucleic Acids Res 1990;18:2835.
12 Weber JL, Kwitek AE, May PE: Dinucleotide repeat polymorphism at the D1S103 locus. Nucleic Acids Res 1990;18:2199.
13 Weber JL, May PE: Dinucleotide repeat polymorphism at the D2S72 locus. Nucleic Acids Res 1990;18:2200.
14 Polymeropoulos MH, Rath DS, Xiao H, Merril CR: Dinucleotide repeat polymorphism at the human preproglucagon gene. Nucleic Acids Res, in press.
15 Brett PM, Melmer G, Gurling HMD: A microsatellite polymorphism at the D3S11 locus. Nucleic Acids Res 1991;19:6978.
16 Weber JL, May PE, Patterson D, Drabkin H, Killary AM: Dinucleotide repeat polymorphism at the D3S196 locus. Nucleic Acids Res 1990;18:4635.
17 HOX 7: Unpublished data from JC Murray, Iowa. In HGM 11 Cytogenet Cell Genet 1991; 58:1322.
18 Weber JL, Kwitek AE, May PE, Killary AM: Dinucleotide repeat polymorphism at D4S174 locus. Nucleic Acids Res 1990;18:4636.
19 Weber JL, May PE: Dinucleotide repeat polymorphism at the D4S171 locus. Nucleic Acids Res 1990;18:2202.
20 Weber JL: D5S208. Genomics, in press.
21 Weber JL, Kwitek AE, May PE: Dinucleotide repeat polymorphisms at the D5S107, D5S108, D5S117 and D5S118 loci. Nucleic Acids Res 1990;18:4035.
22 Mankoo BS, Sherrington R, De La Concha A, Kalsi G, Curtis D, Melmer G, Gurling HMD: Two microsatellite polymorphisms at the D5S39 locus. Nucleic Acids Res 1991;19: 1963.
23 Weber JL: D5S210. Genomics, in press.
24 Litt M, Luty JA: Dinucleotide repeat polymorphism at the D6S89 locus. Nucleic Acids Res 1990;18:4301.
25 Polymeropoulos MH, Rath DS, Xiao H, Merril CR: Tetranucleotide repeat polymorphism at the human coagulation factor XIII. A subunit gene (F13A1). Nucleic Acids Res 1991;19: 4306.
26 Polymeropoulos MH, Rath DS, Xiao H, Merril CR: Trinucleotide repeat polymorphism at the human transcription factor 11D gene. Nucleic Acids Res 1991;19:4307.
27 Weber JL, Kwitek AE, May PE: Dinucleotide repeat polymorphisms at the D7S435 and D7S440 loci. Nucleic Acids Res 1990;18:4039.
28 Weber JL, Kwitek AE, May PE, Patterson D, Drabkin H: Dinucleotide repeat polymorphisms at the D8S85, D8S87 and D8S88 loci. Nucleic Acids Res 1990;18:4038.
29 Weber JL, May PE: Dinucleotide repeat polymorphism at the PENK locus. Nucleic Acids Res 1990;18:2200.
30 Sharma V, Brown D, Smith L, Magenis RE, Litt M: Dinucleotide repeat polymorphism at the D9S55 locus. Nucleic Acids Res 1991;19: 4023.
31 Yuille MAR, Hampson RM, Harris RM, Affara NA, Yates RW, Ferguson Smith MA: CA repeat polymorphism at the ASS locus. Nucleic Acids Res, in press.
32 Decker RA, Moore J, Ponder B, Weber JL: Linkage mapping of human chromosome 10 microsatellite polymorphisms. Genomics 1992;12:604–606.
33 Polymeropoulos MH, Xiao H, Rath DS, Merril CR: Tetranucleotide repeat polymorphism at the human tyrosine hydroxylase gene (TH). Nucleic Acids Res 1991;19:3753.
34 Browne DL, Gault J, Thomspon MB, Hauge XY, Evans GA, Litt M: Dinucleotide repeat polymorphism at the D11S527 locus. Nucleic Acids Res 1991;19:4790.
35 Weber JL, Kwitek AE, May PE: Dinucleotide repeat polymorphisms at the D11S419 and CD3D loci. Nucleic Acids Res 1990;18:4036.
36 Ploos van Amstel HK, Reitsma PL: Tetranucleotide repeat polymorphism in the VWF gene. Nucleic Acids Res 1990;18:4957.
37 Weber JL, Kwitek AE, May PE: Dinucleotide repeat polymorphism at the D13S71 locus. Nucleic Acids Res 1990;18:4638.
38 Weber JL, Kwitek AE, May PE: Dinucleotide repeat polymorphism at the D14S34 locus. Nucleic Acids Res 1990;18:4638.
39 Wang Z, Weber J: Continuous linkage map of human chromosome 14 short tandem repeat polymorphisms. Genomics 1992;13:532–536.
40 Polymeropoulos MH, Rath DS, Xiao H, Merril CR: Tetranucleotide repeat polymorphism at the human c-fes/fps proto-oncogene (FES). Nucleic Acids Res 1991;19:4018.
41 Weber JL, Kwitek AE, May PE: Dinucleotide repeat polymorphisms at the D16S260, D16S261, D16S265, D16S266 and D16S267 loci. Nucleic Acids Res 1990;18:4034.
42 Weber JL, Kwitek AE, May PE, Wallace MR, Collins FS, Ledbetter DH: Dinucleotide repeat polymorphisms at the D17S250 and D17S261 loci. Nucleic Acids Res 1990;18:4640.
43 Iwasaki N, Xiang K, Seino M, Bell GI: Dinucleotide repeat polymorphism at D20S17 (CR1-L127). Nucleic Acids Res 1991;19:6970.
44 Economou EP, Bergen AW, Warren AC, Antonarakis SE: The polydeoxyadenylate tract of Alu repetitive elements is polymorphic in the human genome. Proc Natl Acad Sci 1990;87: 2951–2954.
45 Polymeropoulos MH, Xiao H, Rath DS, Merril CR: Dinucleotide repeat polymorphism at the human cysteine-proteinase inhibitor pseudogene (CSTP). Nucleic Acids Res 1991;19: 1164.
46 Hughes D, Brown J, Hardy J, Chartier-Harlin M-C: A polymorphic dinucleotide repeat in intron 2 of the human cystatin-C gene. Hum Mol Genet 1992;1:143.
47 Polymeropoulos MH, Rath DS, Xiao H, Merril CR: Dinucleotide repeat polymorphism at the human debrisoquine 4-hydroxylase (CYP2D) locus. Nucleic Acids Res 1991;19:1961.
48 Weber JL, May PE: Dinucleotide repeat polymorphism at the D22S156 locus. Nucleic Acids Res 1990;18:4639.

Dementia 1993;4:167–171

L. Edvinsson[a]
L. Minthon[b]
R. Ekman[c]
L. Gustafson[b]

[a] Departments of Internal Medicine and
[b] Psychogeriatrics, University of Lund, and
[c] Department of Psychiatry and Neurochemistry, University of Gothenburg, Sweden

Neuropeptides in Cerebrospinal Fluid of Patients with Alzheimer's Disease and Dementia with Frontotemporal Lobe Degeneration

Key Words
Cerebral spinal fluid
Neuropeptide Y
Somatostatin
Delta sleep-inducing peptide
Vasoactive intestinal peptide
β-Endorphin
Galanin
Antidiuretic hormone
Corticotropin releasing factor
Calcitonin gene-related peptide
Frontal lobe dementia
Dementia of Alzheimer type

Abstract
The two major primary degenerative dementias, dementia of Alzheimer type (DAT) and frontal lobe degeneration of non-Alzheimer type (FLD) have several clinical features in common but also many symptoms that differ. In a clinical material of 80 patients with either of the two forms of dementia (DAT = 39, FLD = 41) we have studied the levels of neuropeptides in the cerebrospinal fluid (CSF) in order to find biochemical markers for CNS affection. The dementia forms were evaluated by careful clinical analysis, psychometric testing and measurement of regional cerebral blood flow. Approximately one third of the subjects died during the completion of the study and neuropathology was performed, confirming the diagnoses. We observed reductions in the CSF levels of antidiuretic hormone and somatostatin in both DAT and FLD. A strong tendency to reduction was noted for neuropeptide Y (NPY). There was a correlation with the duration of disease demonstrating a significant reduction in NPY levels in subjects with DAT. Most notably there was a strong reduction in the levels of delta sleep inducing peptide (DSIP) in DAT cases only. The levels of DSIP in FLD were the same as in controls. The reverse was found for corticotropin releasing factor (CRF) which had a significant reduction in FLD patients but not in those with DAT. The present study indicates a difference in the CSF levels of neuropeptides, observations that these may serve as biochemical markers which differentiate DAT and FLD.

Introduction

Dementia of Alzheimer type (DAT) and frontal lobe degeneration of non-Alzheimer type (FLD) are the most prevalent types of primary degenerative dementia [1, 2]. At present there is no effective way to prevent or ameliorate the progression of these brain diseases. This is partly due to the lack of knowledge of the neurotransmitter involvement in different forms of dementia. DAT has been shown to comprise a reduction of the neurotransmitter acetylcholine and treatment with choline esterase inhibitors has caused some improvement. Recent studies

Prof. Lars Edvinsson
Department of Internal Medicine
University Hospital
S-221 85 Lund (Sweden)

1013-7424/93/0044-0167
$2.75/0

have revealed a beneficial effect of tetrahydroaminoacridin in a subpopulation of DAT [3–7]. The present study was designed to examine and compare a number of neurotransmitters in the cerebral spinal fluid (CSF) of patients with primary degenerative dementia disorders. Several of the neuropeptides such as vasopressin, corticotropin-releasing factor (CRF) and β-endorphin [8] are involved in the discussions related to memory and cognition. In the present study, we have in addition measured CRF, antidiuretic hormone (ADH), β-endorphin, vasoactive intestinal peptide (VIP) and galanin. These neuropeptides were compared to the levels of peptides in dementia previously studied neuropeptide Y (NPY), somatostatin (SOM), and delta sleep-inducing peptide (DSIP) to obtain information whether any of these transmitter systems are affected primarily and if they may differentiate between DAT and FLD.

Materials and Methods

Patients

Eighty patients were included in this study, 39 with DAT and 41 with FLD; age range 35–77 years. The patients were admitted to the psychogeriatric clinic in Lund for examination and treatment of symptoms of dementia. This included psychiatric, neurologic, somatic and laboratory investigations, psychometric testing, regional cerebral blood flow measurements, electroencephalography, and computer tomography. A control group consisted of 11 healthy volunteers (age 23–58 years). None of the controls showed any signs of neurological disorders, dementia or other mental disease according to the clinical judgement.

CSF Samples

CSF samples were removed, following an overnight fast, at 9 a.m. Twelve milliliters of CSF was taken from each patient (the initial 2 ml was discarded) in a sitting position. The CSF sample was mixed and immediately transported in ice water to the laboratory, centrifuged at 1,000 *g* 10 min at +4 °C, divided into 2-ml aliquots in polyethylene vials and stored at –80 °C until assayed.

Radioimmunoassays

For the radioimmunoassay (RIA) of the various peptides, the samples were analyzed in serial dilutions optimized to the linear part of the standard curve and corrected for nonspecific binding. Immunoreactive caltonin gene-related peptide (CGRP) was quantified using a rabbit antiserum (R-8429), raised against synthetic rat CGRP, conjugated to bovine serum albumin, and used in a final dilution of 1:37,500 [9]. Iodinated CGRP was purified by HPLC. This allows measurements of CGRP-like material with a minimum of 2 pmol/l. The interassay variation was 12%. Immunoreactive β-endorphin (BE) was quantified using a rabbit antiserum (K-7762) raised against unconjugated synthetic human BE. The antiserum was used in a final dilution of 1:25,000 and has a negligible cross-reactivity against β-lipotrophin (<1.5%). The detection limit was 10 pmol/l. The interassay coefficient of variation was <10% [10]. Immunoreactive NPY was analyzed as previously described [11]. The antiserum cross-reacted with peptide YY to 33% but not with C-terminal fragments of NPY and PYY. The detection limit was 11 pmol/l and the interassay coefficient of variation was <7%. Immunoreactive SOM was determined using a rabbit antiserum (K18, Milab, Malmö, Sweden) in a final dilution of 1:25,000 [12]. The antiserum does not show cross-reaction with any other known neuropeptides besides cyclic SOM (100%), linear SOM (50%) and (Tyr^1)-SOM (100%). The detection limit was 6 pmol/l, expressed as SOM 15–28 equivalent. The interassay variation was <12%. Immunoreactive somatostatin (SOM) was determined using a rabbit antiserum (K18 Milab, Malmö, Sweden) in a final dilution of 1:25,000. The antiserum does not show cross-reaction with any other known neuropeptides besides cyclic SOM (100%), linear SOM (50%) and Tyr^1)-SOM (100%). The detection limit was 6 pmol/l, expressed as SOM 15-28 equivalent. The interassay variation was <12% [13]. Immunoreactive VIP was determined with a rabbit antiserum (code 7852, Milab, Malmö, Sweden) [14]. The antiserum was used in dilution 1:60,000 and does not cross-react with PHI (peptide histoidine isoleucine), secretin or glucagon. The detection limit was 3 pmol/l, interassay variation 8.5%. Immunoreactive galanin was measured using a specific and sensitive radioimmunoassay [15]. A rabbit antiserum (code No. 8419, Milab) raised against synthetic unconjugated porcine galanin was used in a final dilution of 1:25,000. (^{125}I) Galanin was used as tracer. The detection limit was 10 pmol/l (1 fmol/tube) with 95% confidence. The interassay variation was below 10% in the 15–150 pmol/l range. There was no cross-reactivity of the antibodies with substance P, neurokinin A, or physalaemin up to 1,000 pmol/l.

CRF was measured by a specific RIA using an antihuman (h)CRF serum obtained from a rabbit immunized with synthetic CRF conjugated to bovine serum albumine by glutaraldehyde. ^{125}I-hCRF was prepared by the chloramine T method according to Hunter and Greenwood. The antiserum is directed against the carboxyterminal portion of the antigen and does not cross-react with ovine CRF, hCRF(37–41), hCRF(34–31), ACTH, or β-endorphin. The assay sensitivity is 2 pmol/l and measurements are made directly on unextracted plasma. The interassay variation was below 8% [16]. ADH was measured by the use of a RIA described by Rooke and Baylis [17]. The ADH antiserum was from Dr. P.H. Baylis (The Royal Victoria Infirmary, Newcastle, UK). The antiserum showed little cross-reaction with related peptides (lysine vasopressin <0.03%; arginine vasotocin and oxytocin <0.01%). The limit of detection of plasma ADH after extraction was 1.0 pmol/l and the interassay variation was below 9%.

A highly sensitive RIA for DSIP has been developed at the laboratory [18]. A *p*-hydroxyphenylpropionic acid conjugate of DSIP was used for radioiodination. Using reversed-phase high-performance liquid chromatography the labelled DSIP derivative was isolated in a high yield and with a high specific activity. The assay allows measurement of DSIP-like material with a minimum detectable concentration of 100 pmol/l and an interassay variation expressed as CV below 10%.

Results

Neuropeptides

The results are presented in figures 1–3. The levels of SOM, NPY and DSIP (fig. 1) showed a pattern in accordance with published material: SOM was significantly

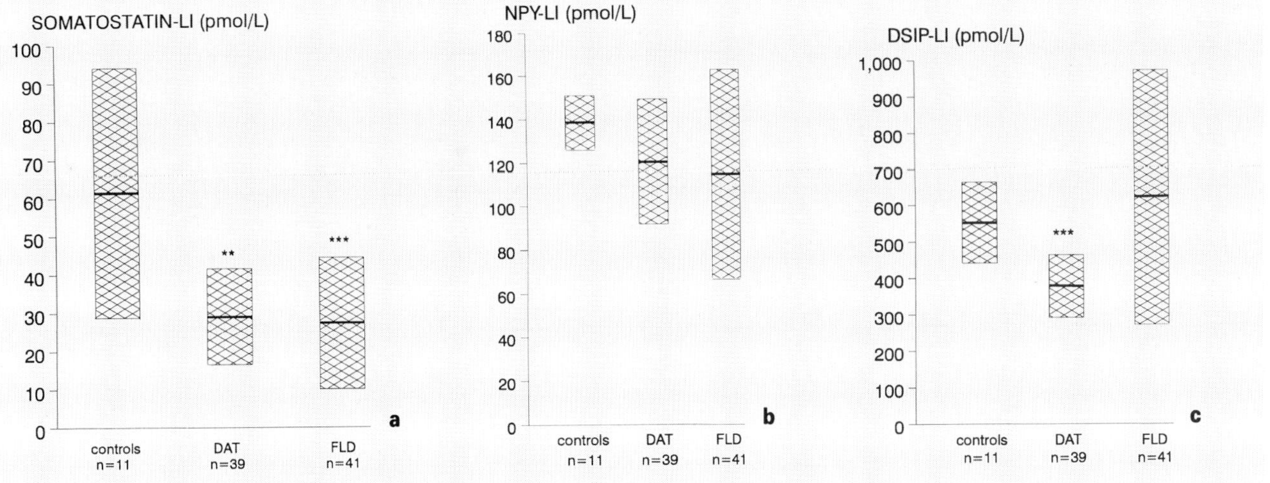

Fig. 1. Somatostatin- (**a**), NPY- (**b**) and DSIP-LI (-like immunoreactivity) (**c**) in controls as compared to DAT and FLD. A significant reduction was seen for SOM-LI (★★ $p < 0.01$, ★★★ $p < 0.001$, Mann-Whitney, Bonferroni correction). For NPY there was no difference between the groups, however, as can be seen the standard deviation was large for DAT and FLD. As noted in results there was a significant correlation with duration of dementia. DSIP-LI was significantly reduced (★★★ $p < 0.001$, Mann-Whitney, Bonferroni correction). Values given represent means ± SD, n represents number of subjects.

reduced in DAT and FLD [19]. NPY reductions were found in both DAT and FLD, but the reduction in this extended material did not reach statistical significant level compared to the relatively small control group of 11 subjects [20]. However, for DAT there was a significant correlation with duration of the disorder (Spearman corr: $p < 0.003$) with lower NPY levels in CSF the longer time the subject has suffered the disease. A correlation with the duration of the disorder was also seen for FLD regardıng the somatostatin concentrations in the CSF (Spearman corr: $p < 0.018$). For DSIP there was a significant reduction for DAT but not for FLD.

For VIP, galanin and β-endorphin there was no significant change in the CSF. Interestingly however, for galanin levels in DAT there was a significant correlation with the duration of disorder, and in this case a slight increase with the year of DAT (Spearman corr: $p < 0.016$). For β-endorphin there was no alteration (fig. 2). In figure 3 the results of ADH, CRF and CGRP are shown. The patterns for these neuropeptides were different. For ADH there was a significantly lower level in both DAT and FLD. Interestingly, both CRF and CGRP showed reduced levels in FLD whereas there were not significant alterations in DAT.

Discussion

A fundamental question for the evaluation of the present findings is whether the clinical diagnosis is correct. The diagnostic procedure was based on the guidelines of Gustafson [21], who described the clinical and neurophysiological criteria of FLD and DAT. The majority of cases have been examined repeatedly and the diagnoses have been confirmed post mortem in deceased cases. An additional important question is the reliability of the methodology for neurotransmitter assessment. To what extent do the neuropeptide levels reflect the degenerative process? The measurement of neuropeptides in the CSF is a problem as to what it reflects. They may represent a summation of a number of facts, may reflect the turnover of neuropeptides in the brain. However, it is clear that patterns emerged which differed between controls and patients with DAT and FLD. The methods used are well characterized and to our knowledge the best methodology available for solving the present task. We have recently carried out HPLC analysis of CSF NPY, SOM and DSIP. The results point towards the presence only of a minor level of the authentic peptides in CSF while most of the examined material represents immuno-

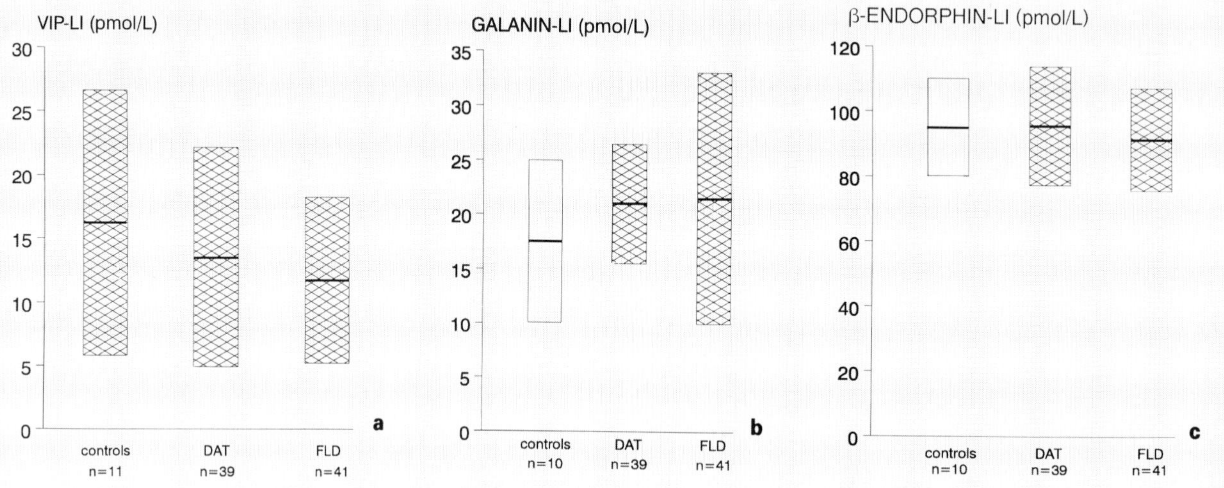

Fig. 2. As can be seen in this figure there was no significant difference in the levels of VIP- (**a**), galanin- (**b**) and β-endorphin-LI (**c**) in the CSF of DAT and FLD as compared to controls or to each other. Values represent means ± SD, n represents number of subjects.

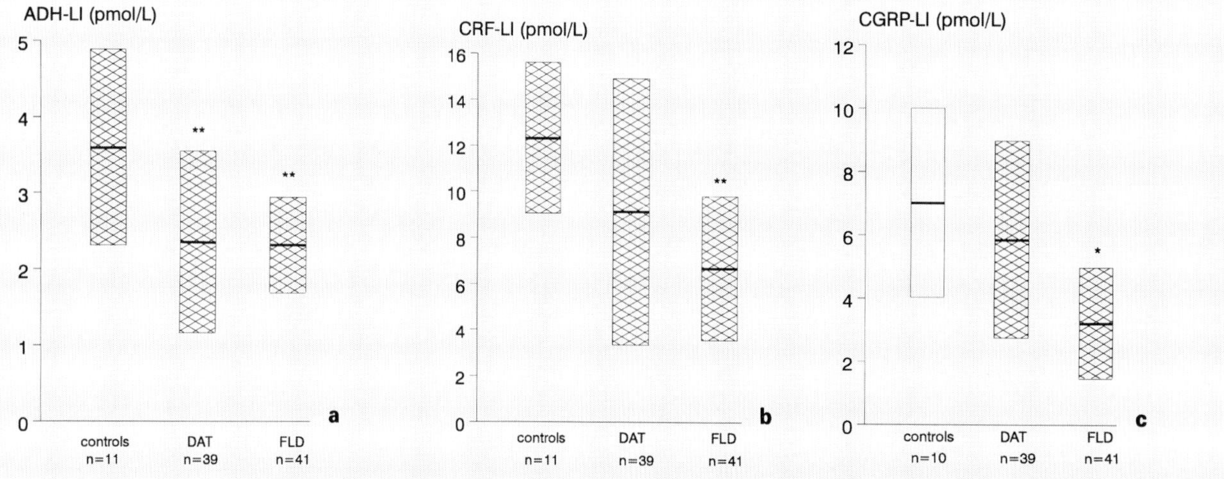

Fig. 3. Concentration of ADH- (**a**), CRF- (**b**) and CGRP-LI (**c**) in the CSF of control for DAT and FLD. Significantly lower levels of AVP(ADH)-LI were seen in both types of organic dementia (★★ $p < 0.01$, Mann-Whitney, Bonferroni correction). For CRF-LI a significant reduction was only seen in FLD (★★ $p < 0.01$). CGRP-LI was slightly reduced in FLD as compared to controls ($p = 0.05$, Kruskal-Wallis). Values represent means ± SD, n represents number of subjects.

reactivity of lower hydrophobicity. The pattern of cortical involvement found in most DAT cases is an accentuation of the degeneration in the temporoparietal association cortex and the temporal-limbic structures [1]. This degenerative pattern is contrary to that found in FLD [22]. FLD is the second most common type of primary degenerative dementia in our catchment area, and found in 8% of a consecutive series of 400 postmortem verified cases. The disease process in FLD affects mainly frontal and anterior temporal regions and to a lesser extent post central cortical areas. The histopathology of DAT and FLD differs in many aspects [22]. The present study is descriptive but it provides a map of neurotransmitter alterations which might provide more insight into the degenerative differences and the possibility to differentiate between DAT and FLD. In DAT there was a significant reduction in ADH, DSIP, and SOM in the CSF. A different pattern of neuropeptide levels in CSF was noted in FLD with reductions in ADH, CRF and SOM compared to DAT. Thus, the similarity is striking, for ADH and SOM the pattern is identical whereas for DSIP the DAT subjects had low levels while the FLD cases had normal levels. In the study of the duration of the disorder, in particular for NPY and SOM, there was a significant correlation with duration. Thus, the more pronounced the DAT subjects the lower the level of these two neuropeptides. One may regard the many neurotransmitters being unaltered in either dementia form as a form of control.

Acknowledgements

We are grateful for the technical assistance of Mrs. Karin Nilsson.

The present study was supported by the Swedish Medical Research Council (grants No. 5958, 07517) and the Medical Faculty, Lund University.

References

1 Brun A, Gustafson L: Distribution of cerebral degeneration in Alzheimer's disease. A clinico-pathological study. Arch Psychiatr Nervenkr 1976;223:15–33.

2 Gustafson L, Brun A, Risberg J: Frontal lobe dementia of non-Alzheimer type; in Wurtman J, et al (eds): Advances in Neurology. Alzheimer's Disease. New York, Raven Press, 1990, vol 51, pp 65-71.

3 Summers WK, Koopmans Summers W, Majovski LV, Marsh GM, Tachiki K, Kling A: Oral tetrahydroaminoacridine in long-term treatment of senile dementia, Alzheimer type. N Engl J Med 1986;315:1241–1245.

4 Minthon L, Gustafson L, Dalfelt G, Hagberg B, Nilsson K, Risberg J, Rosén I, Seiving B, Wendt PE: Oral tetrahydroaminoacridine treatment of Alzheimer's disease evaluated clinically and by regional cerebral blood flow and EEG. Dementia 1993;4:32–42.

5 Nybäck H, Nyman H, Öhman G, Nordgren I, Lindström B: Preliminary experiences and results with THA for the amelioration of symptoms of Alzheimer's disease; in Giacobini E, Becker R (eds): Current Research in Alzheimer Therapy. New York, Taylor & Francis, 1988.

6 Summers WK, Koehler AL, Marsh GM, Tachiki K, Kling A: Long-term hepatotoxicity of Tacrine. Lancet 1989;i:729.

7 Åhlin A, Nybäck H, Junthe T, Öhman G, Nordgren I: Tetrahydroamino acridine in Alzheimer's dementia: Clinical and biochemical results of a double-blind crossover trial. Hum Psychopharmacol 1991;6:109–118.

8 Zager EL, Black PMcL: Neuropeptides in human memory and learning processes. Neurosurgery 1985;17:355–369.

9 Bramnert M, Ekman R, Larsson I, Thorell JI: Characterization and application of a radioimmunoassay for β-endorphin using an antiserum with negligible cross-reactivity against β-lipotropin. Regul Pept 1982;5:65–75.

10 Grunditz T, Ekman R, Håkanson R, Rerup C, Sundler F, Uddman R: Calcitonin gene-related peptide in thyroid nerve fibres and C-cells. Effects on thyroid hormone secretion and response to hypercalcemia. Endocrinology 1986; 119:2313–2323.

11 Widerlöv E, Lindström LH, Wahlestedt C, et al: Neuropeptide Y (NPY) and peptide Y (PYY) as possible cerebrospinal fluid markers for major depression and schizophrenia, respectively. J Psychiatry Res 1988;22:69–79.

12 Wallengren J, Ekman R, Sundler F: Occurrence and distribution of neuropeptides in the human skin. An immunocytochemical and immunochemical study on normal skin and blister fluid from inflamed skin. Acta Derm Venereol 1987;67:185–192.

13 Wallengren J, Ekman R, Sundler F: Occurrence and distribution of neuropeptides in the human skin. An immunocytochemical and immunochemical study on normal skin and blister fluid from inflamed skin. Acta Derm Venereol 1987;67:185–192.

14 Wallengren J, Möller H, Ekman R: Occurrence of substance P, vasoactive intestinal peptide and calcitonin gene-related peptide in factitious and cold urticaria. Arch Dermatol Res 1987;279:512–515.

15 Ekblad E, Arnbjörnsson E, Ekman R, Håkanson R, Sundler F: Neuropeptides in the human appendix, distribution and motor effects. Dig Dis Scl 1989;34:1217–1230.

16 Ekman R, Servenius B, Castro MG, Lowry PJ, Cederlund A-S, Bergman O, Sjögren HO: Biosynthesis of corticotropin releasing hormone in human T-lymphocytes. J Neuroimmunol 1993, in press.

17 Rooke P, Baylis PH: A new sensitive radioimmunoassay for plasma arginine vasopressin. J Immunoassay 1982;3:115–131.

18 Ekman R, Larsson I, Malmquist M, Thorell JI: Radioimmunoassay of delta sleep-inducing peptide using an iodinated *p*-hydroxyphenylpropionic acid derivative as tracer. Regul Pept 1983;6:371–378.

19 Minthon L, Edvinsson L, Ekman R, Gustafson L: Reduced lumbar cerebrospinal fluid somatostatin levels in Alzheimer's disease and dementia with frontotemporal degeneration. Dementia 1991;2:273–277.

20 Minthon L, Edvinsson L, Ekman R, Gustafson L: Cerebrospinal fluid neuropeptide Y-like immunoreactive levels in dementia of Alzheimer type and dementia with frontotemporal degeneration of non-Alzheimer type. Dementia 1990;1:262–266.

21 Gustafson L: Frontal lobe degeneration of non-Alzheimer type I. Clinical picture and differential diagnosis. Arch Gerontol Geriatr 1987;6: 209–223.

22 Brun A: Frontal lobe degeneration of non-Alzheimer type I. Neuropathology Arch Gerontol Geriatr 1987;6:193–208.

Dementia 1993;4:172–177

P.T. Francis
C. Holmes
M.-T. Webster
G.C. Stratmann
A.W. Procter
D.M. Bowen

Miriam Marks Department of Neurochemistry, Institute of Neurology (Queen Square), London, UK

Preliminary Neurochemical Findings in Non-Alzheimer Dementia due to Lobar Atrophy

Key Words
Pick's disease
Dementia of frontal lobe type
Metabolism
Dietary changes
Serotonin
Somatostatin

Abstract
Non-Alzheimer's dementia due to lobar atrophy had choline acetyltransferase activities comparable with control rather than Alzheimer's disease values, based on 3 autopsy proven cases on Pick's disease and biopsies from 3 examples of dementia of frontal lobe type. Muscarinic cholinergic receptors were relatively spared only in Alzheimer's disease. Serotonin receptors were markedly reduced (based on Pick cases) whereas measures that reflected presynaptic serotonergic activity were either not affected or increased. Cerebrospinal fluid and brain tissue measurements suggested that inhibitory interneurones and dopamine release were relatively spared. There was no in vitro evidence of hypometabolism.

Introduction

In studies of patients with primary degenerative dementia, Neary et al. [1] have laid emphasis on the observation that while Alzheimer's disease (AD) is the major cause of widespread social importance, a significant minority of patients do not have this condition. Brun [2], during the neuropathological workup of a large prospective study of 158 dementia cases, found 2.5% had the clear features of Pick's disease and a further 10% appeared to form a separate group without the characteristics of either Pick's disease or AD, and these he called 'frontal lobe degeneration of non-Alzheimer's type'. Although many human post-mortem brain studies of neurodegenerative conditions may be viewed as descriptive, not hypothesis driven research, there was hope that the discovery of neurotransmitter deficiencies would lead to successful treatments. For this reason AD has been the subject of many neurochemical studies, but accurate differentiation between dementing diseases is increasingly important in view of the possibility of therapeutic intervention. The neurochemistry of Pick's disease has been difficult to study, mainly due to the relative rarity of the condition and a lack of suitable tissue. Cummings and Duchen [3] have reviewed 8 autopsy proven cases from this centre. Clinical notes were available in 5 cases. The hemisphere from the brain of one of these was frozen 8 h after death and studied by neurochemical methods (Case 1 [3] and patient aged 68 years [4]). This report describes our preliminary data for non-Alzheimer dementia due to lobar atrophy (LA), which is considered here to include dementia of frontal lobe type (DFLT) [1] and Pick's disease.

Pick's Disease

Three histologically verified post-mortem brains have been studied using neurochemical methods. Patient A was Case 1 of Cummings and Duchen [3], B was AP5 [5] and C, a patient aged 63 [4]. All had swollen cells containing Pick bodies (Pick cells). One probable case (patient D) was also examined. Histological examination of the tem-

Dr. D.M. Bowen
Institute of Neurology
Department of Neurochemistry
1 Wakefield Street
London WC1N 1PJ (UK)

1013–7424/93/0044–0172
$2.75/0

poral lobe from this specimen showed marked shrinkage of the cortex in which there was severe neuronal loss and gliosis. No Alzheimer neurofibrillary tangles were present and no senile plaques were seen. The white matter was heavily gliosed. Although no definite Pick bodies were seen, the distribution of the abnormalities and the absence of neurofibrillary tagles and plaques makes Pick's disease the most likely diagnosis [L.W. Duchen, pers. commun.].

In Pick's disease, brain choline acetyltransferase (ChAT) activity was higher than those of AD samples and comparable to control value. Presynaptic 'serotonergic' activities were higher than AD and control values, except for one measure in patient D (table 1) [data for patient B is given in ref. 5]. By contrast, muscarinic cholinergic receptors and binding of ligands that reflect 5-HT_1 receptors were lower in Pick's disease (table 2, 3). Muscarinic binding was not reduced in the frontal cortex [6]. Both

Table 1. ChAT and 'serotonergic' activities of temporal lobe

Patients		ChAT, nmol/min/g protein	5-HT + 5-HIAA µg/g protein
Pick's disease	A	46	10.8
	C	64	13.1
	D[a]	38	5.5
C (n = 10–16)		55 ± 4	5.8 ± 0.6
AD (n = 7–8)		21 ± 4[b]	7.5 ± 0.7

5-HT and 5-HIAA identifies serotonin and major metabolite; C identifies control ± SEM.
a No specific histological changes.
b Significant difference from AD.
Methods as described in Bowen et al. [28].

Table 2. Ligand binding to temporal lobe

Patients		Binding, pmol/lobe		
		LSD	β-adrenergic	muscarinic
Pick's disease	A	382	86	849
	C	420	139	1,060
	D[a]	347	214	491
C (7)		1,364 ± 165	207 ± 106	1,986 ± 587
AD (7)		673 ± 203[b]	227 ± 55	1,758 ± 377

Values are means ± SD.
a No specific histological changes.
b Significant difference from AD.
Methods as described im Bowen et al. [28].

Table 3. Serotonin and glutamate receptors

Receptor		Pick's disease (patient B)	AD (n = 9)	Depressive pseudodementia (n = 1)	Other (n = 4)
$5HT_{1A}$	1 nM	7.9	12.6 ± 4.5	12.5	15.1 ± 4.7
	4 nM	12.5	20.0 ± 7.3	20.8	23.7 ± 6.6
5-HT_2	0.5 nM	9.3	8.8 ± 2.0	9.3	10.8 ± 5.4
	2 nM	26.1	23.5 ± 6.7	18.2	20.9 ± 7.9
NMDA complex	1	0.17	0.10 ± 0.02	0.10	0.09 ± 0.01
	2	0.20	0.16 ± 0.03	0.17	0.15 ± 0.03
	3	0.35	0.40 ± 0.11	0.51	0.36 ± 0.05
Pyramidal neurones					
Supragranular		30	27 ± 7	44	42 ± 14
Infragranular		30	31 ± 7	44	32 ± 11

NMDA identifies N-methyl-*D*-aspartic acid.
Data is for the superior frontal cortex expressed as fmol/mg protein or number of cells/field ± SD.
1, 2 and 3 identify [^{3}H]-MK801 binding without added amino acids, plus glutamate and glutamate plus glycine, respectively (a DFLT case had values for 1, 2 and 3 of 0.13, 0.14 and 0.25, respectively).
Methods as described in Procter et al. [17, 31] and Middlemiss et al. [30].

Table 4. Concentration of DA metabolite and interneurone marker in ventricular fluid

Patient groups	HVA pmol/ml	SLI fmol/ml
DFLT	1,168 ± 188 (4)	25, 34 (2)
Intractable depression	1,444 ± 106 (35)	ND
AD	1,190 ± 159 (8)	29 ± 12 (8)
Other neurological	985 ± 49 (8)	25 ± 21 (15)

Values are means ± SEM; ND = not determined.
Methods as described in Francis et al. [32, 33].

Table 5. Frontal cortex: index DFLT case compared with AD

	DFLT % control	AD % control	
ChAT activity	112	37[b]	(21;20)
5-HT conc.	200[a]	78	(9;25)
5-HT release	34 [130, 478]	51[b]	(6;6)
NA release	18 [63, 91]	74	(5;6)
DA release	92 [67, 593]	192	(5;6)
5HIAA conc.	116	63[b]	(9;26)
SLI conc.	149	151	(4;17)
SLI release	142 [142, 156]	129	(6;7)
ASP conc.	76[a]	119[b]	(3;16)
GABA conc.	102	144	(3;14)
O_2 uptake	149[a] [147[a]]	109	(5;7)

Conc. = tissue concentration; release, K^+ (50 m*M*) evoked from tissue prisms; uptake by homogenates. Numbers in parentheses identify numbers of AD and control samples. Numbers in brackets identify other cases. [Methods as described in ref. 5, 32, 34–37.]
[a] Outside control range (± 2 SD).
[b] Significant values versus DFLT.

Table 6. Cholinergic marker in frontal cortex

Patient group	ChAT activity nmol/min/100 mg protein
DFLT (3)	10.2 ± 3.2
AD (17)	3.7 ± 4.0*
C (20)	10.3 ± 1.0

Values are mean ± SD.
* $p < 0.01$ compared with control (C).
Methods as described in Palmer et al. [35].

supragranular and infragranular pyramidal cell counts in frontal cortex were comparable to AD values in patient B (table 3). Yet binding of radioligand to the $5HT_{1A}$ receptor, proposed to be located on these cells [7], was lower.

β-Amyloid precursor protein (β-APP) immunoreactivity was determined by western blotting in fractions of superior frontal cortex from 15 of the rapidly chilled brains collected promptly post-mortem (table 3) [5]. No correlations of any β-APP species with coma duration or other demographic features were observed. Supragranular pyramidal neurone counts (see table 3) related to amount of one β-APP species (negative and positive correlations for supernant and particulate fractions, respectively, prepared and analyzed using methods similar to those of Arai et al. [8] and the Pick's disease count predicted the β-APP value (patient B).

Dementia of Frontal Lobe Type

Lumbar and ventricular fluid and cortical biopsy tissue has been studied from patients diagnosed according to Neary et al. [1]. In DFLT cerebrospinal fluid values for 5-HIAA, homovanillic acid (HVA), and 3-methyoxy-4-hydroxyphenylglycol (MHPG) were similar to those for other groups of patients, including controls (fig. 1; table 4) [not all data is shown]. Table 5 shows that the mean release values for 5-HT and dopamine (DA) were high (214 and 250% of control, respectively). The noradrenaline (NA) release value of at least the index DFLT case was low (table 5) [9]. Somatostatin-like immunoreactivity (SLI) was low in only lumbar fluid (fig. 2, table 4) while tissue concentration and release values were higher than control (table 5). At the end point of disease tissue, values may be low as has been found in AD [10, 11]. Ventricular fluid glutamate values were similar to those of other patients while for aspartate (ASP) the values tended to be among the highest [data not shown]. There was no evidence of either hypometabolism (based on O_2 uptake, table 5) or reduced ChAT activity (table 6).

Discussion

The main finding of this study was that patients with LA had ChAT-specific activities comparable with control rather than AD values [6, 11–13]. Thus LA seemed to differ from AD and 'related' disorders ('Lewy body' and 'mixed senile and vascular dementia') as there was no evidence of obvious and selective presynaptic cholinergic pathology in LA [14, 15]. On balance there is also no evidence for loss of other ascending cortical innervation in LA. Most data suggested that in LA presynaptic serotonergic activity was either not affected or increased [13]. Tissue release in vitro and cerebrospinal fluid data suggested that DA release in vivo was not significantly affected.

LA and AD both showed biochemical evidence of relative sparing of inhibitory cortical interneurones, based on the data for SLI [6, 16], GABA and the 5-HT_2 receptor, proposed to be located on these cells [7, 17]. By contrast [^{3}H]lysergic acid diethylamide (LSD) binding to 5-HT receptors (predominantly not to 5-HT_2 receptors) is markedly reduced based in the Pick cases [13]. Relative sparing of interneurones and DA was also a feature of AD [16] so LA and AD share these biochemical characteristics.

Behavioural symptoms in dementia may be a manifestation of underlying structural brain damage, and have been considered as important socially as the cognitive dysfunction [18]. The behavioural symptoms of AD have been considered analogous to the Kluver-Bucy behavioural syndrome which follows temporal lobectomy in monkeys [19]. However while the prevalence of the various components of this syndrome in dementia shows an intercorrelation and association with temporal lobe atrophy, 'binge-eating' appears to occur in the absence of the other components [19, 20], perhaps therefore with an independent aetiology. All patients with Pick's disease considered by Commings and Duchen [3] showed oral/dietary changes early in the disease. For example, patient A began 'eating massive amounts of apples' and 'later radically changed his diet – eating large quantities of cottage cheese and yogurt', and the other 4 cases they described 'ate anything in reach' (Case 2), 'always returned punctually for tea' (Case 3), was 'noted to overstuff his mouth with food – stole food' (Case 4) and 'would eat anything on the table' (Case 5). These observations are of interest as LSD, used to assess 5-HT receptors in table 2, is a potent 5-HT_{1C} receptor agonist [29] and antagonists at this site increase feeding [21, 22], suggesting that the abnormality of this site in Pick's disease underlies this particular symptom.

Preliminary Implications for Pharmacotherapy

Lack of evidence for hypometabolism in either LA or AD (table 5) suggested that cortical tissues did not have a reduced capacity for energy metabolism. Thus reduced neuronal activity (due to neuronal degeneration) proba-

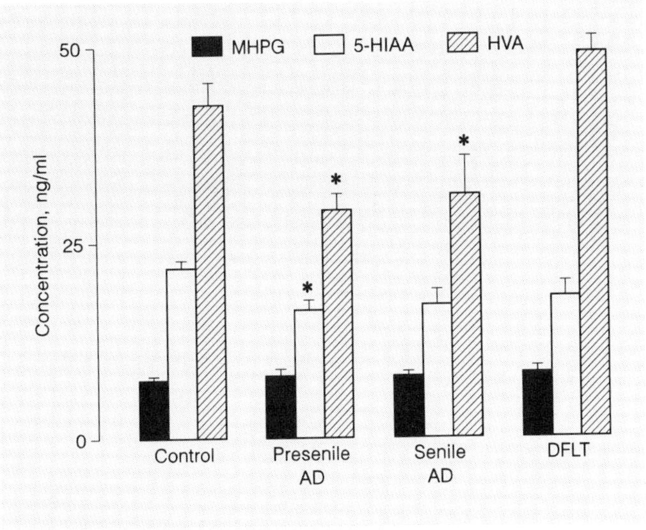

1

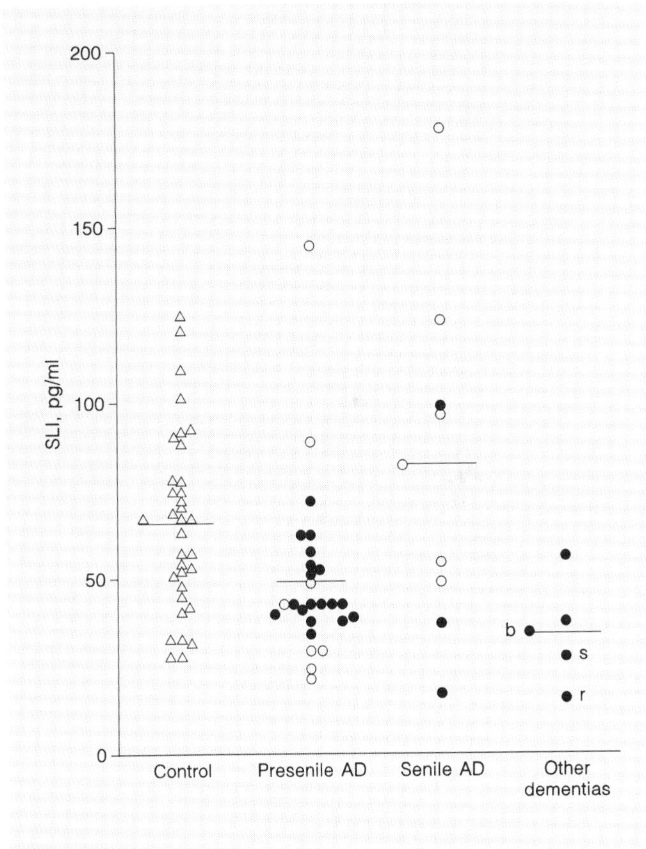

2

Fig. 1. Monoamine metabolites in 3 patients with DFLT and control and presenile Alzheimer patients (24–26 and 28–35, respectively). The senile Alzheimer group (>70 years) contains 9 or 10 patients. Bars represent SEM. * Results significantly different from control ($p < 0.05$, ANOVA-LSD; after Palmer and Bowen [38].

Fig. 2. SLI concentration in individual samples of lumbar fluid, DFLT cases are identified by letter. The filled-in circles identify 'drug-free' patients. The horizontal lines represent the mean value for each group; after Francis et al. [39].

bly explains, at least in part, in vivo hypometabolism [23, 24]. LA and AD showed biochemical evidence of relative sparing of cortical interneurones. By contrast, glutamatergic cortical pyramidal neurones have been most difficult to study but histological methods suggested that in circumscribed areas these degenerate in both disorders [16, 25, 26]. Muscarinic receptors were relatively spared only in AD (table 2) [27] and LSD binding was more affected in LA than AD. This suggested that inadvertent inclusion of LA in clinical trials will complicate interpretation. However, lumbar fluid SLI determination may provide an exclusion criterion.

In summary these preliminary neurochemical findings highlight some interesting differences between LA and AD. Further more detailed investigations should improve understanding of the relationship between DFLT and Pick's disease.

Acknowledgements

Drs. M.J. Goodhardt, P. Milner (nee White), A.M. Palmer, S.L. Lowe and N.R. Sims kindly carried out some of the determinations. We are also grateful to the many people involved in the collection and classification of human samples in particular Dr. R.O. Barnard, Dr. R. Doshi, Professor L.W. Duchen and Professor D. Neary.

The research was supported by Astra Arcus, Brain Research Trust ('Miriam Marks Department'), Medical Research Council and Sir Halley Stewart Trust.

References

1 Neary D, Showden JS, Northen B, Goulding P: Dementia of frontal lobe type. J Neurol Neurosurg Psychiatry 1988;51:353–361.
2 Brun A: Frontal lobe degeneration of non-Alzheimer type 1. Neuropathology. Arch Gerontol Geriatr 1987;6:193–208.
3 Cummings JL, Duchen LW: Kluver-Bucy Syndrome in Pick disease: Clinical and pathologic correlations. Neurology 1981;31:1415–1422.
4 White P, Hiley CR, Goodhardt MJ, Carrasco LH, Keet JP, Williams IE, Bowen DM: Neocortical cholinergic neurons in elderly people. Lancet 1977;i:668–671.
5 Procter AW, Palmer AM, Francis PT, Lowe SL, Neary D, Murphy E, Doshi R, Bowen DM: Evidence of glutamatergic denervation and possible abnormal metabolism in Alzheimer's disease. J Neurochem 1988;50:790–802.
6 Wood PL, Etienne P, Lat S, Nair NPV, Finlayson MH, Gauthier SG, Palo J, Haltia M, Paetau P, Bird ED: A post-mortem comparison of the cortical cholinergic system in Alzheimer's disease and Pick's disease. J Neurol Sci 1983;62:211–217.
7 Francis PT, Pangalos MN, Pearson RCA, Middlemiss DN, Stratmann GC, Bowen DM: 5-HT_{1A} but not 5-HT_2 receptors are enriched on neocortical pyramidal neurones destroyed by intrastriatal volkensin. J Pharmacol Exp Ther 1992;261:1273–1281.
8 Arai H, Lee VM-Y, Messinger ML, Greenberg BD, Lowery DE, Trojanowski JQ: Expression patterns of β-amyloid precursor protein (β-APP) in neural and nonneural human tissues from Alzheimer's disease and control subjects. Ann Neurol 1991;30:686–693.
9 Luque JM, Chan-Palay V: Alterations in tyrosine hydroxylase immunoreactive neurons of the locus ceruleus in Pick's disease. Dementia 1991;2:291–296.
10 Francis PT, Pangalos MN, Bowen DM: Animal and drug modelling for Alzheimer synaptic pathology. Prog Neurobiol 1992;39:517–545.
11 Dickson DW, Horoupian DS, Thal LJ, Davies P, Walkley S, Terry RD: Kluver-Buchy syndrome and amyotrophic lateral sclerosis: A case report with biochemistry, morphometrics, and golgi study. Neurology 1986;36:1323–1329.
12 Bowen DM, Benton JS, Spillane JA, Smith CCT, Allen SJ: Choline acetyltransferase activity and histopathology of frontal neocortex from biopsies of demented patients. J Neurol Sci 1982;57:191–202.
13 Sparks DL, Markesbery WR: Altered serotonergic and cholinergic synaptic markers in Pick's disease. Arch Neurol 1991;48:796–799.
14 Bowen DM, Davison AN: Biochemical studies of nerve cells and energy metabolism in Alzheimer's disease. Br Med Bull 1986;42:75–80.
15 Perry EK, Kerwin JM, Perry RH, Irving D, Blessed G, Fairbairn AF: Cerebral cholinergic activity is related to the incidence of visual hallucinations in senile dementia of Lewy body type. Dementia 1990;1:2–4.
16 Bowen DM: Treatment of Alzheimer's disease: Molecular pathology versus neurotransmitter-based therapy. Br J Psychiatry 1990;157:327–330.
17 Procter AW, Lowe SL, Palmer AM, Francis PT, Esiri MM, Stratmann GC, Najlerahim A, Patel AJ, Hunt A, Bowen DM: Topographical distribution of neurochemical changes in Alzheimer's disease. J Neurol Sci 1988;84:125–140.
18 Procter AW, Francis PT, Stratmann GC, Bowen DM: Serotonergic pathology is not widespread in Alzheimer patients without prominent aggressive symptoms. Neurochem Res 1992;17:917–922.
19 Burns A, Jacoby R, Levy R: Psychiatric phenomena in Alzheimer's disease. IV: Disorders of behaviour. Br J Psychiatry 1990;157:86–94.
20 Hope RA, Fairburn CG, Goodwin GM: Increased eating in dementia. Int J Eating Disord 1989;8:111–115.
21 Dourish CT, Clark ML, Fletcher A, Iversen SD: Evidence that blockade of postsynaptic 5-HT_1 receptor elicits feeding in satiated rats. Psychopharmacology 1989;97:54–58.
22 Kennett GA, Curzon G: Potencies of antagonists indicate that 5-HT_{1C} receptors mediate mCPP-induced hypophagia. Br J Pharmacol 1991;103:2016–2020.
23 McGeer EG, McGeer PL, Kamo H, Tago H, Harrop R: Cortical metabolism, acetylcholinesterase staining and pathological changes in Alzheimer's disease. Can J Neurol Sci 1986;13:511–516.
24 Goldstein S, Reivich M: Cerebral blood flow and metabolism in aging dementia. Clin Neuropharmacol 1991;14(suppl 1):S34–S44.
25 Neary D, Snowden JS, Mann DMA, Northen B, Goulding PJ, Macdermott N: Frontal lobe dementia and motor neurone disease. J Neurol Neurosurg Psychiatry 1990;53:23–32.
26 Mann DMA, South PW, Snowden JS, Neary D: Dementia of frontal lobe type: Neuropathology and immunohistochemistry. J Neurol Neurosurg Psychiatry, in press.
27 Weinberger DR, Gibson R, Coppola R, Jones DW, Molchan S, Sunderland T, Berman KF, Reba RC: The distribution of cerebral muscarinic acetylcholine receptors in vivo in patients with dementia. A controlled study with ^{123}IQNB and single photon emission computed tomography. Arch Neurol 1991;48:169–176.

28 Bowen DM, Allen SJ, Benton JS, Goodhardt MJ, Haan EA, Palmer AM, Sims NR, Smith CCT, Spillane JA, Esiri MM, Neary D, Snowden JS, Wilcock GK, Davison AN: Biochemical assessment of serotonergic and cholinergic dysfunction and cerebral atrophy in Alzheimer's disease. J Neurochem 1983;41: 266–272.
29 Burris KD, Breeding M, Sanders-Bush E: (+)Lysergic acid diethylamide, but not its nonhallucinogenic congeners, is a potent serotonin 5-HT_{1C} receptor agonist. J Pharmacol Exp Ther 1991;258:891.
30 Middlemiss DN, Palmer AM, Edel N, Bowen DM: Binding of the novel serotonin agonist 8-hydroxy-2-(di-n-propylamino)tetralin in normal and Alzheimer brain. J Neurochem 1986; 46:993–996.
31 Procter AW, Stramann GC, Francis PT, Lowe SL, Bertolucci PHF, Bowen DM: Characterisation of the glycine modulatory site of the N-methyl-*D*-aspartate receptor-ionophore complex in human brain. J Neurochem 1991;56: 299–310.
32 Francis PT, Bowen DM, Lowe SL, Neary D, Mann DM, Snowden JS: Somatostatin content and release measured in cerebral biopsies from demented patients. J Neurol Sci 1987;78:1–16.
33 Francis PT, Pangalos MN, Stephens PH, Bartlett JR, Bridges PK, Malizia AL, Neary D, Procter AW, Thomas DJ, Bowen DM: Antemortem measurements of neurotransmission: Possible implications for pharmacotherapy of Alzheimer's disease and depression. J Neurol Neurosurg Psychiatry, 1993;56:80–84.
34 Francis PT, Poynton A, Lowe SL, Najlerahim A, Bridges PK, Bartlett JR, Procter AW, Bruton CJ, Bowen DM: Brain amino acid concentrations and Ca^{2+}-dependent release in intractable depression assessed antemortem. Brain Res 1989;494:315–324.
35 Palmer AM, Francis PT, Benton JS, Sims NR, Mann DM, Neary D, Snowden JS, Bowen DM: Presynaptic serotonergic dysfunction in patients with Alzheimer's disease. J Neurochem 1987;48:8–15.
36 Palmer AM, Francis PT, Bowen DM, Benton JS, Neary D, Mann DM, Snowden JS: Catecholaminergic neurones assessed ante-mortem in Alzheimer's disease. Brain Res 1987;414: 365–375.
37 Lowe SL, Bowen DM, Francis PT, Neary D: Ante mortem cerebral amino acid concentrations indicate selective degeneration of glutamate-enriched neurons in Alzheimer's disease. Neuroscience 1990;38:571–577.
38 Palmer AM, Bowen DM: Neurochemical approaches to cognitive disorders; in Lister RG, Weingartner HJ (eds): Perspectives on Cognitive Neuroscience. Oxford, Oxford University Press, 1991, pp 436–466.
39 Francis PT, Bowen DM, Neary D, Palo J, Wikstrom J, Olney J: Somatostatin-like immunoreactivity in lumbar cerebrospinal fluid from neurohistologically examined demented patients. Neurobiol Aging 1984;5:183–186.

Dementia 1993;4:178–185

John Collinge
Mark S. Palmer

Prion Disease Group, Department of Biochemistry and Molecular Genetics, St. Mary's Hospital Medical School, London, UK

Prion Diseases in Humans and Their Relevance to Other Neurodegenerative Diseases

Key Words
Prions
Degenerative brain disease
Molecular genetics
Immunoblotting

Abstract
Molecular genetics has led to considerable advances in our understanding of the transmissible spongiform encephalopathies. The identification of pathogenic mutations in the prion protein gene has enabled a molecular reclassification of the familial forms of these diseases, which may now be referred to as inherited prion diseases. Prion diseases of both humans and animals are associated with deposition of an abnormal isoform of a host-encoded protein, the prion protein (PrP). Human prion diseases have inherited, sporadic and acquired forms. A considerable body of evidence now supports the idea that the transmissible agent in these diseases may be an abnormal isoform of the prion protein. The identification of pathogenic mutations in the PrP gene has enabled the identification of cases of inherited prion disease that would not have been recognised using existing clinical and pathological diagnostic criteria. Since marked clinical and neuropathological overlap between the different neurodegenerative disorders is well recognised, PrP gene analysis is of increasing importance in differential diagnosis. Frontal lobe dementia of non-Alzheimer type and Pick's disease share a number of important clinical and pathological features with prion diseases, and could be considered as candidate prion diseases. However, we have not been able to demonstrate either PrP mutations or the presence of the disease-associated isoform of prion protein in several well-characterised families with these disorders.

Introduction

The transmissible spongiform encephalopathies or prion diseases are a group of neurodegenerative diseases which affect both humans and animals. They have traditionally been known as the transmissible spongiform encephalopathies or slow virus diseases since they can be transmitted by inoculation from one host to another (of the same or different species) following extremely long incubation periods, and because they demonstrate similar histological features including widespread 'spongiform' vacuolation of the brain. The first disease of this group to be recognised was scrapie, a naturally occurring disease of sheep and goats [1]. Transmissible mink encephalopathy and chronic wasting disease of mule deer and elk, along with bovine spongiform encephalopathy (BSE), are dis-

John Collinge
Prion Disease Group
Department of Biochemistry and Molecular Genetics
St. Mary's Hospital Medical School
London W2 1PG (UK)

1013–7424/93/0044–0178
$2.75/0

eases of farmed animals and have probably arisen from the inclusion of scrapie-contaminated material in the production of protein supplements which have been fed to these and other captive animals. Recently described spongiform encephalopathies of both domestic cats and various zoo animals have probably also arisen from contaminated foodstuffs carrying the transmissible agent. BSE has developed to epidemic proportions in British cattle (with over 2,000 cows per month being affected) and this has resulted in considerable public concern that there may be a risk to human health from ingestion of BSE contaminated tissues.

The human diseases have been classically described as Creutzfeldt-Jakob disease (CJD), Gerstmann-Sträussler syndrome (GSS) and kuru. CJD classically presents as a rapidly progressive dementia usually with myoclonus and often with extrapyramidal, cerebellar and pyramidal signs. Atypical types of CJD are, however, well recognised. The condition is rapidly progressive and most patients die within 12 months of onset. Routine investigations are unhelpful with the exception of the electroencephalogram (EEG), which sometimes shows characteristic pseudoperiodic sharp wave activity. Patients are afebrile throughout the clinical course and there are no inflammatory or immunological markers of infection. Detailed epidemiological studies [2] show a random distribution of cases without the clustering expected for an infectious disease (with 3 exceptions which will be addressed later). However, most importantly 5–15% of cases occur in a familial context. GSS, by contrast, is classically regarded as a chronic cerebellar ataxia, dementia occurring later in a much more prolonged clinical course. GSS is nearly always familial, and, like the familial forms of CJD, shows an autosomal dominant pattern of segregation in these families. Kuru, a disease principally involving a progressive ataxia, affected the Fore linguistic group of Papua New Guinea and was spread by ritualistic endocannibalism [3]. The disease has now almost disappeared although a few cases are still reported resulting from the long incubation period of the disease.

Both the animal and human diseases share common histological features. The classic triad of spongiform change, astrocytic proliferation and neuronal loss may be accompanied by the deposition of amyloid as plaques [4]. Multicentric plaque formation is the pathological hallmark of GSS. These plaques consist principally of an abnormal isoform of a host-encoded protein (prion protein) discussed below. Diffuse staining with antisera to the prion protein where amyloid plaques are not apparent is reported in experimental scrapie in mice [5] and may be present in human cases [6].

All these diseases are transmissible to experimental animals by intracerebral innoculation. Kuru was successfully transmitted to the chimpanzee in 1966 [7]. Transmission of CJD followed in 1968 [8]. GSS was also experimentally transmitted to animals in 1981 [9]. These diseases are not, however, contagious and case to case spread in humans has only occurred via rather unusual routes. Such 'iatrogenic CJD' cases have resulted from the use of inadequately sterilised intracerebral electrodes, dura mater and corneal grafting and from use of cadaveric pituitary-derived human growth hormone and gonadotrophin [10].

The potential risk to human health from BSE has highlighted this group of diseases but they have been an intense area of interest for some time because of the unique features of the transmissible agent. Prusiner [11] coined the term 'prion' in 1982 to distinguish the transmissible agent from viruses. All the prion diseases are associated with the accumulation in the brain of an abnormal, partially protease-resistant, isoform of a host-encoded protein, the prion protein or PrP [12]. The normal cellular isoform of the protein is designated PrP^{C} and the disease-related isoform PrP^{Sc}. Both PrP^{C} and PrP^{Sc} are encoded by the same single copy gene and the entire coding sequence is contained within a single open reading frame offering no potential for the production of multiple splice products. Direct studies of both PrP^{C} and PrP^{Sc} have shown no amino acid differences between them. The difference is therefore assumed to result from an as yet unidentified post-translational modification [13]. PrP^{C} is a cell surface sialoglycoprotein of unknown function highly conserved across mammalian species and expressed in most tissues [14].

Attempts to enrich brain fractions for infectivity lead to the production of purified fractions consisting essentially of the disease-related isoform of the prion protein. Such fractions can transmit the disease to experimental animals and extensive attempts to demonstrate co-purification of significant nucleic acids have been unsuccessful [15, 16]. The infectivity of such fractions is remarkably resistant to agents that would inactivate nucleic acids such as nucleases and ultraviolet irradiation [12]. Such work has led to the suggestion that the infective agent may be devoid of nucleic acid and may consist essentially of an abnormal form of PrP.

As has been mentioned, 5–15% of CJD cases occur in a familial context and GSS is usually familial, and in both cases an autosomal dominant pattern of segregation is seen [17]. The prion protein gene, mapped in humans to the short arm of chromosome 20, was an obvious candi-

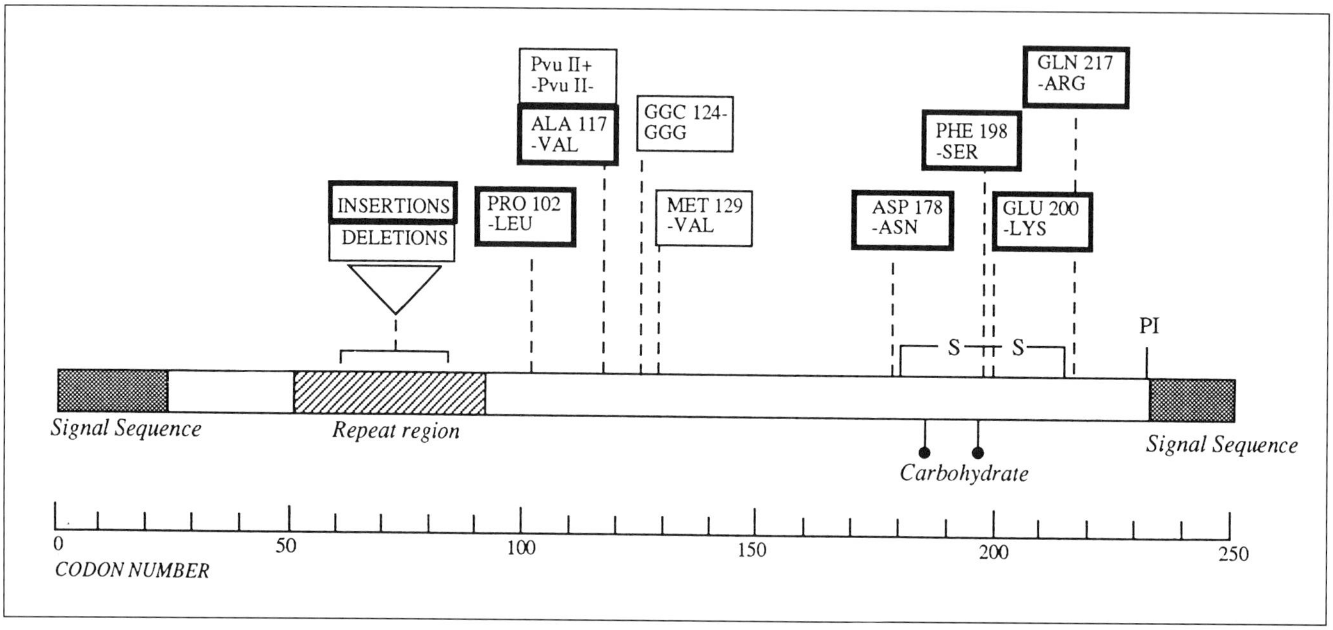

Fig. 1. Prion protein gene open reading frame identifying all the currently recognised mutations and polymorphisms by codon number (this is identical to amino acid residue number). Pathogenic mutations seen in inherited prion diseases are indicated in heavy boxes; polymorphisms are indicated in lighter boxes. Insertions of 4, 5, 6, 7, 8, or 9 additional copies of an octapeptide repeat are associated with disease while deletions of a single octarepeat represent an uncommon polymorphic variation seen in the normal population. An internal disulphide bond and the position of carbohydrate attachment are indicated. The signal sequences are cleaved during maturation of the protein and a phosphatidyl inositol anchor (PI) added at the new carboxy terminal.

date gene. The demonstration of genetic linkage between a missense variant in the PrP gene and GSS demonstrated that GSS is an autosomal dominant Mendelian disorder, in addition to being transmissible to experimental animals by inoculation [18]. These diseases are therefore biologically unique in being both inherited and infectious. Furthermore, this mutation, which results in a proline to leucine substitution in the prion protein, has now been demonstrated in a number of families with GSS from several countries but is absent from normal controls suggesting that it was a pathogenic mutation. The pathogenicity of this missense codon 102 mutation was directly demonstrated by the finding that transgenic mice encoding an analogous mutation spontaneously developed spongiform neurodegeneration [19].

An extensive family of PrP gene mutations have now been reported by various workers in affected individuals from kindreds with CJD/GSS (fig. 1) [14]. These dramatic advances in the molecular genetics of the human diseases and their subsequent transgenic modelling in mice have now led to the prion diseases becoming the best understood group of neurodegenerative conditions.

Inherited Prion Diseases

A map of the currently recognised PrP mutations and polymorphisms is given in figure 1. The identification of such genetic markers has led to the possibility of molecular diagnosis of cases which are not classical of the CJD or GSS phenotype. The first application of such diagnosis by DNA analysis enabled a case thought on clinical grounds to be suffering from Alzheimer's disease to be re-classified as GSS [20]. Further screening of neurodegenerative cases using prion protein gene analysis resulted in the identification of several further families with a 144 base pair insertion mutation, none of which were previously thought to be CJD or GSS. Thus the availability of direct gene tests has enabled molecular diagnosis of cases of inherited prion disease thought on clinical grounds to be suffering from other neurodegenerative illnesses such as Alzheimer's disease, Huntington's disease, Pick's disease or Parkinsonism [21]. Indeed 1 case, with an extremely prolonged dementing/ataxic illness, at autopsy had none of the characteristic features of CJD or GSS (or indeed of any specific neurodegenerative disease) [22]. This case raised the possibility that these diseases were underdiagnosed since a considerable proportion of dementia patients at autopsy do not show diagnostic histological features and additionally questioned the usefulness of the term 'spongiform encephalopathy' as a generic name for these diseases. Further studies demonstrated that these families were related and formed a large kindred which demonstrated marked phenotypic heterogeneity [21, 23]. While an affected individual in this family had a rapidly progressive clinical course characteristic of CJD other affected family members have had a much longer duration GSS type illness. Histological features vary from classical spongiform encephalopathy (with or without prion protein immunoreactive amyloid plaques) to a complete absence of histological features of spongiform encephalopathy or other defined neurodegenerative diseases [22]. Such findings have led to the realisation that familial CJD and GSS are parts of a spectrum of what seems more sensibly called inherited prion disease. Such intrafamilial phenotypic heterogeneity (revealed in particular when cases are ascertained by genetic screening rather than by studying cases already ascertained on the basis of their characteristic clinicopathological features), is now being appreciated in the other inherited prion diseases. The recent identification of mutations in the beta amyloid precursor protein gene on chromosome 21 in several unrelated families with early onset Alzheimer's disease as well as in the phenotypically distinct hereditary cerebral haemorrhage with amyloidosis Dutch type will also contribute towards such a rational, aetiological re-classification of neurodegenerative diseases hitherto largely classified by a range of clinical and morphological criteria [21]. A family in which both Alzheimer type dementia and haemorrhagic infarction cases are found has now been described [25]. It remains to be seen if other such 'APP-opathies' will be uncovered.

The recent report of a PrP mutation in two families with what is described as fatal familial insomnia [26] further emphasises that the availability of genetic markers allows us to search for the actual phenotypic range of expression of these diseases, overcoming the selection bias of studying only cases ascertained using existing criteria.

The identification of a missense mutation at codon 200 of the PrP gene [27] has resulted in an explanation for the 3 well-known ethnogeographic clusters of CJD referred to earlier [28, 29]. There has been an unexplained 100-fold higher prevalence of CJD in Slovakia and amongst Libyan Jews and an additional large cluster of cases in Chile. With respect to the Libyan Jewish focus this had previously been attributed to dietary habits including eating lightly cooked sheep brain and sheep eyeballs. It is now known that all 3 clusters are familial and that all affected individuals have the codon 200 mutation. This variant of inherited prion disease shows incomplete penetrance in that the mutation has been described in apparently unaffected elderly family members [28, 30].

The identification of a novel PrP mutation in the so-called Indiana kindred of GSS has been of particular interest since in addition to the presence of prion protein immunoreactive plaques in this family there are also marked neurofibrillary tangles which are morphologically and antigenically indistinguishable from those seen in Alzheimer's disease [14]. This might suggest that neurofibrillary tangles are a relatively non-specific finding as they can result from both mutations in the PrP gene and APP gene.

This availability of direct gene tests for inherited prion diseases allows pre-symptomatic and antenatal testing for these markers. The genetic counselling problems closely resemble those in HD and pre-symptomatic testing after careful counselling has been described [31].

Sporadic and Iatrogenic Prion Disease

More than 85% of CJD occurs as a sporadic illness of unknown aetiology. In addition rare cases have been caused by iatrogenic contamination. Human prion diseases therefore have inherited, sporadic and acquired types. Acquired types include these iatrogenic cases resulting from accidental inoculation with the disease agent and kuru, transmitted by cannibalism. Iatrogenic routes include the use of inadequately sterilised intracerebral electrodes, dura mater and corneal grafting and from the use of human cadaveric pituitary-derived growth hormone and gonadotrophin. It is of interest that while iatrogenic cases following intracerebral inoculation with the transmissible agent clinically resemble classical sporadic CJD, those cases resulting from peripheral inoculation with the agent resemble kuru, and present primarily as an ataxic illness.

In the UK 1,908 individuals were treated with pituitary-derived growth hormone and 6 have subsequently developed CJD [32]. Each batch of hormone had been pooled from up to 3,000 glands and each iatrogenic case had received material from more than one batch. No single batch could be implicated in all the cases. Therefore it was conceivable that most and possibly all these patients had been exposed to some level of the infective agent and therefore that these individuals who went on to develop CJD may represent a genetically susceptible population. We felt that such a group may be the most appropriate to study for evidence of genetic susceptibility to prion diseases in humans. We screened all 7 UK cases of CJD arising from the use of pituitary-derived hormones (6 growth hormone related and 1 gonadotrophin related) for PrP gene variations including a coding polymorphism at codon 129 (either methionine or valine being encoded). We found that a significant excess (4/7) were homozygous for the less common PrP valine 129 allele [33]. Population frequencies for this polymorphism in Caucasians were estimated as 37% Met/Met, 51% Met/Val and 12% Val/Val based on a sample size of 106.

On the basis that PrP valine 129 homozygotes may be genetically susceptible to prion diseases, at least following inoculation, we examined a group of known sporadic CJD cases. If they too resulted from environmental exposure to prions, we might expect to find a similar excess of valine 129 homozygotes. We did not find such an excess but found that all but 1 of 22 cases were homozygotes either for Met or Val [34]. The single heterozygote turned out, on further enquiry to have a family history of dementia and may not have been a sporadic case. The implications of these results are discussed below in the context of a general model for prion diseases.

Whether a broad range of both clinical and histological presentation will also be found with sporadic and iatrogenic prion disease, as seen with the inherited forms, remains to be established. A case of sporadic CJD with characteristic clinical features but lacking histological features has been transmitted to experimental animals [Prusiner, personal communication]. Although transmission studies have in the past been attempted with a wide range of neurodegenerative conditions, it could be that cases with less typical histology are more difficult to transmit.

Relevance to Degeneration of Frontal Lobe Type

Marked phenotypic overlap, at least as regards clinical features, is apparent between the prion diseases and many other neurodegenerative conditions. The demonstration of the existence of cases of inherited prion diseases entirely lacking the diagnostic histological features of spongiform encephalopathies also raises the possibility that some other conditions may turn out to be variants of prion disease in their entirety or, more likely, that some cases currently classified as other neurodegenerative conditions may turn out to be prion diseases. In the case of for instance Parkinson's disease, amyotrophic lateral sclerosis, Huntington's disease or Alzheimer's disease, instances of misdiagnosis on clinical grounds of inherited prion diseases as these conditions have already been reported but clearly only in a very small minority of cases. However with, for example, frontal lobe degeneration of non-Alzheimer type (FLD) or Pick's disease (PD), these could be plausibly considered as candidate prion diseases. Frontal lobe features are well recognised in at least one type of inherited prion disease [21]; Pick type cells have been reported in CJD [35]. We have therefore studied several well documented families with FLD (in collaboration with Drs Brun and Gustafson) and PD (in collaboration with Drs Bakker, Roos and Groen) using both direct sequencing of the PrP gene and immunoblotting techniques. No prion protein mutations were detected and immunoblotting of CNS tissue revealed no protease resistant PrP [Collinge et al., in preparation]. It therefore seems likely that the core diseases currently described as FLD and Pick's are not prion diseases according to present criteria. However the possibility of non-coding mutations in the PrP gene or that the tissue sampled for PrP^{Sc} may have been from an area with little disease cannot be excluded, although tissue samples used for immunoblotting studies in the case of FLD were taken from the frontal pole where histological changes are most apparent. Transmission experiments should still be attempted.

Nature of the Infective Agent

The finding that transgenic mice encoding the corresponding mutation to that seen in one form of human inherited prion disease spontaneously develop spongiform neurodegeneration established the pathogenicity of this, and by association, the other human mutations [19]. The combination of the powerful linkage data with this transgenic modelling clearly demonstrates the central role of PrP in the aetiology of these diseases. A further support to the hypothesis that an abnormal isoform of PrP is the infective agent (or at least its key constituent) would be provided by demonstration that brain tissue from such transgenically modified, spontaneously ill mice could transmit the disease to other animals. Such data has now been presented [36] and its full publication is awaited with interest.

An unresolved issue in the prion diseases is the finding of different 'strains' of the transmissible agent in the murine scrapie model. There are distinct scrapie isolates which produce distinct incubation times and pathology in the same host. The existence of a large number of strains of the transmissible agent is difficult to explain in terms of a protein only model, although the actual number of defined strains remains controversial. Weissmann [37] has recently proposed a hypothetical model which seeks to reconcile the existence of strain diversity with a protein only model of transmissibility. He argues that PrP^{Sc} may associate with a nucleic acid ('co-prion') which while not essential for infectivity confers the phenotypic variability associated with the different strains. According to such a model, the strain characteristics, but not the transmissibility, would be lost following treatment with agents which inactivate nucleic acids. A direct test of this model is awaited.

Prion Protein Sequence Homology and a Model of Prion Replication

Transgenic approaches have provided advances in the understanding of the so-called 'species barrier' in prion diseases. Although the disease can be transmitted from one species to another by inoculation, such transmission occurs typically only in a small proportion of inoculated animals and usually only after prolonged incubation periods. Prusiner et al. [38] constructed transgenic mice which, in addition to expressing normal murine PrP, overexpressed normal hamster PrP. Such transgenic animals became fully susceptible to hamster-derived infective agent with incubation periods which were inversely proportional to the level of hamster PrP expression. The species barrier was therefore ablated by the introduction of PrP from the same species as the inoculum. Furthermore, when such mice were inoculated with mouse-derived infective agent they produced infectivity which could be readily transmitted to wild type mice but not to hamsters. Conversely, when such transgenic mice were inoculated with hamster-derived prions, they produced infectivity which was fully pathogenic for hamsters but not for mice. One interpretation of this data is that a direct interaction between homologous PrP molecules may be involved, at some stage, in the disease process. The idea is that a direct interaction between PrP^{Sc} and PrP^{C} occurs with the formation of a dimer or more complex interaction and that PrP^{Sc} serves to catalyse a conformational (or other post-translational) change in PrP^{C} to convert it to PrP^{Sc} [38, 39]. This could then result in a chain reaction which would lead to the progressive accumulation of the protease resistant PrP^{Sc}. This accumulation presumably leads to the disease state.

Our findings that sporadic CJD occurs predominately in individuals homozygous with respect to the coding polymorphism at codon 129 provides strong support for this type of model. Heterozygotes are partially protected against developing a prion disease since the protein protein interaction would presumably be less favoured between heterologous molecules. Additional evidence in this regard is provided by the finding that in a large kindred with inherited prion disease (with a 144 base pair insertion in the PrP gene) affected individuals who are also heterozygous at codon 129 die at a significantly later age than those who are homozygotes at this codon [40].

The implication from the codon 129 genotype studies in the human diseases is that for optimum progression of this process the interacting proteins need to be homologous. Heterozygosity at codon 129, which may protect against the development of human prion diseases, can be seen as a sort of internal 'species barrier' [34]. The idea that a protein in an abnormal conformation may drive the normal protein into the abnormal conformation is not unprecedented. Such a situation has been described for the p53 protein where wild type and mutant proteins have different conformations and co-translation of both proteins drives the wild type protein into the mutant conformation [41].

According to this model prion diseases arise as a result of inoculation with PrP^{Sc} which then sets off the chain reaction or, in the inherited forms, mutant PrP may spontaneously undergo the conversion to PrP^{Sc} and then trigger the disease as before. The aetiology of sporadic CJD is undetermined. The epidemiological studies suggest a random process. It seems most likely that these cases arise either from somatic mutation (with the subsequent spontaneous development of PrP^{Sc} in the clone of cells expressing one of the pathogenic mutations), or from spontaneous conversion of PrP^{C} into PrP^{Sc} as a rare event [34].

As different proteins, presumably valine 129 PrP and methionine 129 PrP will differ slightly in their propensity to undergo the transformation from PrP^{C} to PrP^{Sc}. Therefore valine 129 PrP molecules may be more susceptible to the conformational (or other post-translational) change when they meet PrP^{Sc}. This would account for the excess of valine 129 PrP homozygotes amongst iatrogenic cases [33].

We have recently reported preliminary findings on 8 cases of clinically suspected CJD (referred to the UK CJD epidemiological surveillance study) which were heterozygous at polymorphic codon 129. Two of these cases had made a clinical recovery and were not CJD, one case was typical CJD (and confirmed neuropathologically), however the remaining 4 cases were all clinically atypical cases with long duration illness. This suggests that 'atypical CJD' may represent the occurrence of sporadic disease in a codon 129 heterozygote [42].

Since inherited prion disease cases are necessarily heterozygous with respect to the pathogenic mutation, it may be that this explains some of the phenotypic difference between sporadic disease and the usually much more prolonged illness in inherited cases. 'GSS' may represent prion disease occurring in a heterozygote, while CJD occurs in individuals with complete PrP sequence homology.

Conclusions

The study of the human familial diseases has provided gene markers enabling a re-assessment of their phenotypic range and the realisation that the conditions previously identified as spongiform encephalopathies were part of a spectrum of disease. This work has also provided decisive evidence for the central role of the prion protein in these diseases. The new terminology of prion diseases not only provides a rational aetiological classification of these conditions but underlines the importance of examining previous schemes of classification of neurodegenerative disease. With respect to FLD, it seems that the classical syndrome does not appear to be a variant of prion disease although the clear clinicopathological overlap of FLD and inherited prion diseases should encourage a search for PrP gene mutations in all such familial cases.

These breakthroughs in our understanding of the human prion diseases have now opened up powerful transgenic approaches to understanding the molecular mechanisms of prion replication. It is now clear that a modified form of prion protein itself is the central, and possibly the sole, constituent of the transmissible agent. The model of prion replication discussed does not challenge fundamental biological principles although it clearly remains unprecedented as a disease mechanism. The conformational change hypothesis suggests that drugs with selective binding properties for PrP^{Sc} might be expected to inhibit the disease process and such ligands could provide rational therapies for the human diseases.

References

1 McGowan JP: Scrapie in sheep. Scott J Agric 1922;5:365–375.
2 Brown P, Cathala F, Raubertas RF, Gajdusek DC, Castaigne P: The epidemiology of Creutzfeldt-Jakob disease: Conclusion of a 15-year investigation in France and review of the world literature. Neurology 1987;37:895–904.
3 Alpers M: Epidemiology and clinical aspects of kuru; in Prusiner SB, McKinley MP (eds): Prions: Novel Infectious Pathogens Causing Scrapie and Creutzfeldt-Jakob Disease. San Diego, Academic Press, 1987, pp 451–465.
4 Beck E, Daniel PM: Neuropathology of transmissible spongiform encephalopathies; in Prusiner SB, McKinley MP (eds): Prions: Novel Infectious Pathogens Causing Scrapie and Creutzfeldt-Jakob Disease. San Diego, Academic Press, 1987, pp. 331–385.
5 Bruce ME, McBride PA, Farquhar CF: Precise targeting of the pathology of the sialoglycoprotein, PrP, and vacuolar degeneration in mouse scrapie. Neurosci Lett 1989;102:1–6.
6 Lantos PL, McGill IS, Janota I, Doey LJ, Collinge J, Bruce MT, Whatley SA, Anderton BH, Clinton J, Roberts GW, Rossor MN: Prion protein immunocytochemistry helps to establish the true incidence of prion diseases. Neurosci Lett 1992;147:67–71.
7 Gajdusek DC, Gibbs CJ, Alpers M: Experimental transmission of a kuru-like syndrome to chimpanzees. Nature 1966;209:794–796.
8 Gibbs CJ, Gajdusek DC, Asher DM, Alpers MP, Beck E, Daniel PM, Matthews WB: Creutzfeldt-Jakob disease (spongiform encephalopathy): Transmission to the chimpanzee. Science 1968;161:388–389.
9 Masters CL, Gajdusek DC, Gibbs CJ Jr: Creutzfeldt-Jakob disease virus isolations from the Gerstmann-Sträussler syndrome with an analysis of the various forms of amyloid plaque deposition in the virus-induced spongiform encephalopathies. Brain 1981;104:559–588.
10 Weller RO: Iatrogenic transmission of Creutzfeldt-Jakob disease. Psychol Med 1989;19:1–4.
11 Prusiner SB: Novel proteinaceous infectious particles cause scrapie. Science 1982;216:136–144.
12 Prusiner SB: Prions and neurodegenerative diseases. N Engl J Med 1987;317:1571–1581.
13 Stahl N, Baldwin MA, Teplow D, Hood L, Beavis R, Chait B, Gibson BW, Burlingame AL, Prusiner SB: Cataloging post-translational modifications of the scrapie prion protein by mass spectrometry; in Prusiner SB, Collinge J, Powell J, Anderton B (eds): Prion Diseases of Humans and Animals. London, Ellis Horwood, 1992.
14 Prusiner SB: Molecular biology of prion diseases. Science 1991;252:1515–1522.
15 Meyer N, Rosenbaum V, Schmidt B, Gilles K, Mirenda C, Groth D, Prusiner SB, Riesner D: Search for a putative scrapie genome in purified prion fractions reveals a paucity of nucleic acids. J Gen Virol 1991;72:37–49.
16 Riesner D, Kellings K, Meyer N, Mirenda C, Prusiner SB: Nucleic acids and scrapie prions; in Prusiner SB, Collinge J, Powell J, Anderton B (eds): Prion Diseases of Humans and Animals. London, Ellis Horwood, 1992.
17 Masters CL, Harris JO, Gajdusek DC, Gibbs CJ, Bernoulli C, Asher DM: Creutzfeldt-Jakob disease: patterns of worldwide occurrence and the significance of familial and sporadic clustering. Ann Neurol 1979;5:177–188.
18 Hsiao K, Baker HF, Crow TJ, Poulter M, Owen F, Terwilliger JD, Westaway D, Ott J, Prusiner SB: Linkage of a prion protein missense variant to Gerstmann-Sträussler syndrome. Nature 1989;338:342–345.
19 Hsiao KK, Scott M, Foster D, Groth DF, DeArmond SJ, Prusiner SB: Spontaneous neurodegeneration in transgenic mice with mutant prion protein. Science 1990;250:1587–1590.

20 Collinge J, Harding AE, Owen F, Poulter M, Lofthouse R, Boughey AM, Shah T, Crow TJ: Diagnosis of Gerstmann-Sträussler syndrome in familial dementia with prion protein gene analysis. Lancet 1989;ii:15–17.

21 Collinge J, Brown J, Hardy J, Mullan M, Rossor MN, Baker H, Crow TJ, Lofthouse R, Poulter M, Ridley R, Owen F, Bennett C, Dunn G, Harding AE, Quinn N, Doshi B, Roberts GW, Honavar M, Janota I, Lantos PL: Inherited prion disease with 144 base pair gene insertion: II Clinical and pathological features. Brain 1992;115:687–710.

22 Collinge J, Owen F, Poulter M, Leach M, Crow TJ, Rossor MN, Hardy J, Mullan MJ, Janota I, Lantos PL: Prion dementia without characteristic pathology. Lancet 1990;336:7–9.

23 Poulter M, Baker HF, Frith CD, Leach M, Lofthouse R, Ridley RM, Shah T, Owen F, Collinge J, Brown J, Hardy J, Mullan M, Harding AE, Bennett C, Doshi B, Crow TJ: Inherited prion disease with 144 base pair gene insertion: I: Genealogical and molecular studies. Brain 1992;115:675–685.

24 Hardy J, Mullan M, Chartier-Harlin MC, Brown J, Goate A, Rossor M, Collinge J, Roberts G, Luthert P, Lantos P, Naruse S, Kaneko K, Tsuji S, Miyatake T, Shimizu T, Kojima T, Nakano I, Yoshioka K, Sakaki Y, Miki T, Katsuya T, Ogihara T, Roses A, Pericak-Vance M, Haan J, Roos R, Lucotte G, Favid F: Molecular Classification of Alzheimer's disease. Lancet 1991;337:1342–1343.

25 Hendriks L, van Duijn CM, Cras P, Cruts M, Van Hul W, van Harskamp F, Warren A, McInnis MG, Antonarakis SE, Martin J-J, Hofman A, Van Broeckhoven C: Presenile dementia and cerebral haemorrhage linked to a mutation at codon 692 of the β-amyloid precursor protein gene. Nature Genet 1992;1:218–221.

26 Medori R, Tritschler H-J, LeBlanc A, Villare F, Manetto V, Ying Chen H, Xue R, Leal S, Montagna P, Cortelli P, Tinuper P, Avoni P, Mochi M, Baruzzi A, Hauw JJ, Ott J, Lugaresi E, Autilio-Gambetti L, Gambetti P: Fatal familial insomnia, a prion disease with a mutation at codon 178 of the prion protein gene. N Engl J Med 1992;326:444–449.

27 Goldgaber D, Goldfarb LG, Brown P, Asher DM, Brown WT, Lin S, Teener JW, Feinstone SM, Rubenstein R, Kascsak RJ, et al: Mutations in familial Creutzfeldt-Jakob disease and Gerstmann-Sträussler-Scheinker's syndrome. Exp Neurol 1989;106:204–206.

28 Goldfarb LG, Mitrova E, Brown P, Toh BK, Gajdusek DC: Mutation in codon 200 of scrapie amyloid protein gene in two clusters of Creutzfeldt-Jakob disease in Slovakia. Lancet 1990;336:514–515.

29 Goldfarb LG, Korczyn AD, Brown P, Chapman J, Gajdusek DC: Mutation in codon 200 of scrapie amyloid precursor gene linked to Creutzfeldt-Jakob disease in Sephardic Jews of Libyan and non-Libyan origin. Lancet 1990; 336:637–638.

30 Hsiao K, Meiner Z, Kahana E, Cass C, Kahana I, Avrahami D, Scarlato G, Abramsky O, Prusiner SB, Gabizon R: Mutation of the prion protein in Libyan Jews with Creutzfeldt-Jakob disease. N Engl J Med 1991;324:1091–1097.

31 Collinge J, Poulter M, Davis MB, Baraitser M, Owen F, Crown TJ, Harding AE: Presymptomatic detection or exclusion of prion protein gene defects in families with inherited prion diseases. Am J Hum Genet 1991;49:1351–1354.

32 Buchanan CR, Preece MA, Milner RD: Mortality, neoplasia, and Creutzfeldt-Jakob disease in patients treated with human pituitary growth hormone in the United Kingdom. BMJ 1991;302:824–828.

33 Collinge J, Palmer MS, Dryden AJ: Genetic predisposition to iatrogenic Creutzfeldt-Jakob disease. Lancet 1991;337:1441–1442.

34 Palmer MS, Dryden AJ, Hughes JT, Collinge J: Homozygous prion protein genotype predisposes to sporadic Creutzfeldt-Jakob disease. Nature 1991;352:340–342.

35 Clarke AW, Manz HJ, White CJ, Lehmann J, Miller D, Coyle JT: Cortical degeneration with swollen chromatolytic neurons: its relationship to Pick's disease. J Neuropathol Exp Neurol 1986;45:268–284.

36 Hsiao KK, Groth D, Scott M, Yang SL, Serban A, Rapp D, Foster D, Torchia M, DeArmond SJ, Prusiner SB: Genetic and transgenetic studies of prion proteins in Gerstmann-Sträussler-Scheinker disease; in Prusiner SB, Collinge J, Powell J, Anderton B (eds): Prion Diseases of Humans and Animals. London, Ellis Horwood, 1992.

37 Weissmann C: A 'unified theory' of prion propagation. Nature 1991;352:679–683.

38 Prusiner SB, Scott M, Foster D, Pan KM, Groth D, Mirenda C, Torchia M, Yang SL, Serban D, Carlson GA, et al: Transgenetic studies implicate interactions between homologous PrP isoforms in scrapie prion replication. Cell 1990;63:673–686.

39 Weissmann C: Spongiform encephalopathies. The prion's progress. Nature 1991;349:569–571.

40 Baker HF, Poulter M, Crow TJ, Frith CD, Lofthouse R, Ridley RM, Collinge J: Amino acid polymorphism in human prion protein and age at death in inherited prion disease. Lancet 1991;337:1286.

41 Milner J, Medcalf EA: Cotranslation of activated mutant p53 with wild type drives the wild type p53 protein into the mutant conformation. Cell 1991;65:765–774.

42 Collinge J, Esmonde TFG, Campbell T, Will RG, Palmer MS: Homozygous prion protein genotype as a marker for sporadic Creutzfeldt-Jakob disease. Am J Hum Genet 1992;51:A32.

Dementia 1993;4:186–187

Jarl Risberg
Ulla Passant
Siegbert Warkentin
Lars Gustafson

Department of Psychogeriatrics,
University Hospital, Lund, Sweden

Regional Cerebral Blood Flow in Frontal Lobe Dementia of Non-Alzheimer Type

Key Words
Regional cerebral blood flow
Frontal lobe dementia
133-Xenon inhalation method

Abstract
Twenty-five out of 26 cases of autopsy-verified frontal lobe degeneration of non-Alzheimer type (FLD) were found to have focal frontal or frontotemporal blood flow reductions involving both hemispheres. The deviant case had an asymmetric frontal pathology only apparent on the right side. Focal reduction of blood flow in the frontal lobes is, however, a common and unspecific flow abnormality found in e.g. Pick's disease, Creutzfeldt-Jakob's disease, and in some cases of Alzheimer's disease. Low frontal flow has also been reported in schizophrenia and in toxic encephalopathy. Since a characteristic feature of FLD is a steady progress of the pathology, serial flow measurements extending over several years are especially informative.

The dysfunction of frontal and fronto-temporal areas which clinically is evident in frontal lobe degeneration of non-Alzheimer type (FLD) can be imaged with methods for measurement of the regional cerebral blood flow (rCBF). The interpretation of rCBF changes in FLD as reflections of cortical functional changes is based on the finding of preserved coupling between cortical function, metabolism and blood flow in dementia [1, 2]. Most of our patients with autopsy-verified diagnosis of FLD have been studied with the xenon-133 inhalation method using multiple stationary scintillation detectors [3–5]. Nine such patients were described in the proceedings of the first FLD conference in Lund in 1986 [6] and all were shown to have focal frontal flow diminutions in addition to a subnormal global flow level. Serial measurements in these patients showed the expected accentuation of the flow pathology with clinical progress. It was also clear from this investigation that similar frontal flow diminutions could be seen in other dementing disorders. Four patients with neuropathological diagnosis of Pick's disease showed focal decreases with the same regional distribution as the FLD cases. The pathology in the Pick cases was even more accentuated than in FLD, especially in later stages of the disorder. This investigation also included some other patients with clinical symptoms of frontal lobe dysfunction but with other diagnoses than FLD and Pick's disease at autopsy. Two cases of Creutzfeldt-Jakob's disease were found to have frontal flow pathology and this was also found in two patients with Alzheimer's disease. The Alzheimer patients had, however, parieto-temporal flow decreases in addition to the frontal pathology and could thus be distinguished from the FLD patients, who had no focal pathology in posterior areas. A case of thalamic infarct showed also focal frontal flow decreases but the severity of the pathology varied with no evident progress over a time span of 18 months. A characteristic feature of this functional cortical disturbance, likely to be caused by the subcortical lesion, is thus a greater variability over time compared to disorders with primary cortical involvement.

It was concluded from this study that patients with the diagnosis of FLD always had focal frontal flow decreases but that this was an unspecific sign shared with several other conditions with frontal lobe dysfunction. In the present study the material from 1986 has been updated with additional patients who at autopsy were diagnosed as cases of FLD.

Jarl Risberg, PhD
CBF Laboratory
Department of Psychogeriatrics
University Hospital
S–221 85 Lund (Sweden)

1013–7424/93/0044–0186
$2.75

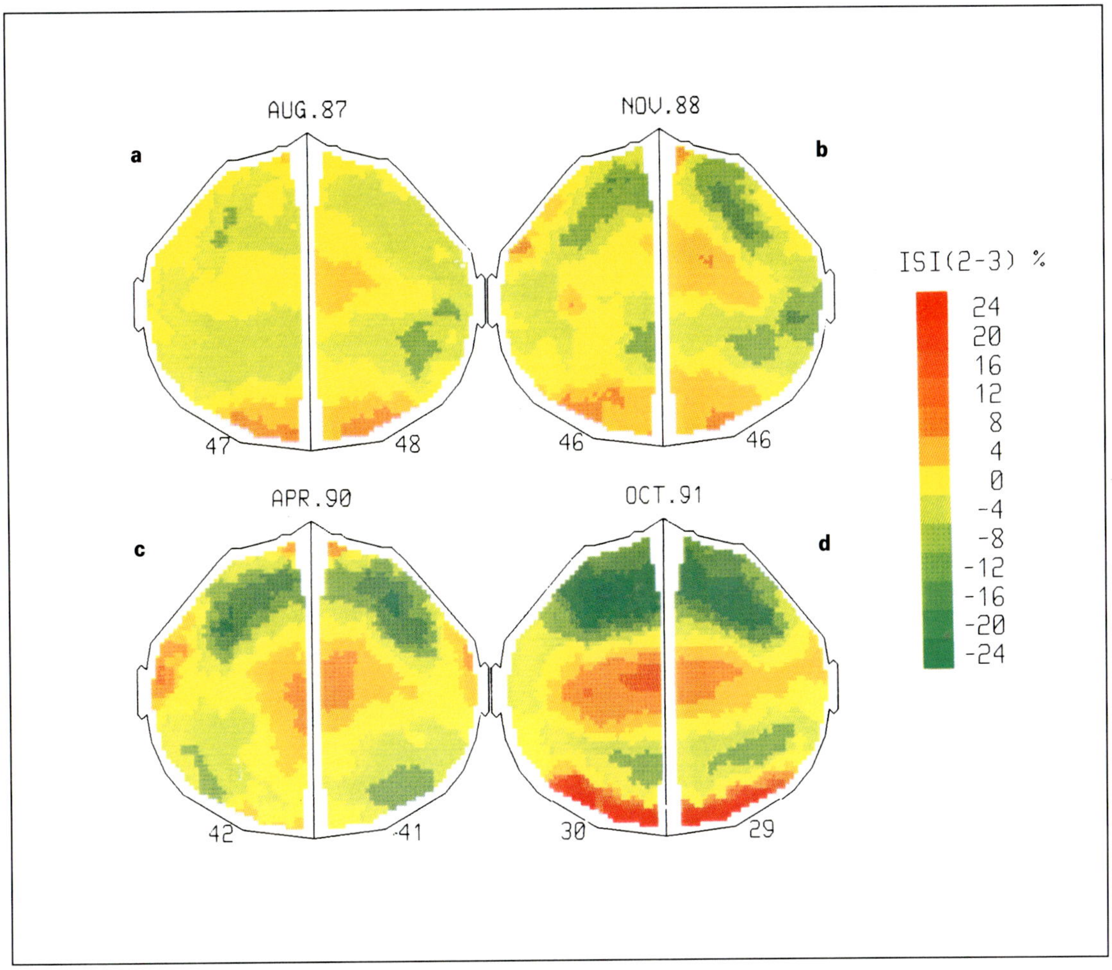

Fig. 1. Four measurements of the regional cerebral blood flow (rCBF) in a patient with clinical signs of frontal lobe dementia. The measurements were made by the xenon-133 inhalation method and a high-resolution recording device with stationary detectors (Cortexplorer). The hemispheric means are shown in the lower part of each flow map and regional variations above (red) or below (green) this mean are indicated by the colour code.

a A female patient who at the age of 61 became unconcentrated, anxious, apathetic and failed at work. When she was investigated one year later (August 87), she showed lack of insight, perseveration, moderate amnesia but had preserved orientation. The rCBF level was normal but the flow distribution was pathologic with slight decreases in frontal areas.

b (November 88). The patient displayed emotional unconcern and social neglect and the frontal focal flow decreases were more pronounced.

c (April 90). The patient was restless with memory failure and semimutism. The mean rCBF level had decreased by 11% with further accentuation of the frontal pathology.

d (October 91). The clinical picture was dominated by mutism, amimia, aggressiveness, hyperphagia and auditory hallucinations. She was, however, still capable of writing her name and knew her date of birth. The rCBF measurement showed a further decrease of the mean flow level and very pronounced frontal flow pathology.

Material and Methods

Material

The present group constitutes a part of a larger material of 150 deceased patients presented elsewhere [7]. In these patients, rCBF results were available together with an autopsy-based dementia diagnosis. For the present study, 26 patients with an FLD diagnosis at autopsy and 4 additional patients in whom the rCBF pathology was interpreted (erroneously) as indicating FLD were selected.

Methods

The neuropathological diagnosis was based on the criteria described by Brun [8]. The rCBF was measured by the 133-xenon inhalation method [3, 4] either using a 32-detector equipment or a high-resolution system with 254 probes (Cortexplorer 256 HR, Scan. Detectronic Inc, Hadsund, Denmark). The technical features of the system and the measurement procedure have been described in detail elsewhere [5, 9].

The result of the rCBF investigation was interpreted by visual inspection of the flow pattern evaluating its deviation from normative data [10]. The pattern assumed to indicate FLD had to be dominated by bilateral focal frontal flow decreases with relatively preserved posterior areas.

Results

The 26 patients with the diagnosis of FLD at autopsy were in all cases but one diagnosed as FLD by rCBF. The deviant case had frontal flow pathology but with a focal decrease only on the right side. This asymmetry was interpreted as indicating cerebrovascular disorder. Three cases with an erroneous rCBF diagnosis of FLD were found to have Alzheimer's disease with frontal flow diminutions most likely caused by incomplete white matter infarcts [SIWI; 11] located mainly anteriorly. One case with frontal cerebral infarcts was evaluated as a case of FLD on the basis of the rCBF pattern.

Discussion

It is evident from the present findings that the frontal dysfunction in FLD is accompanied by substantial focal frontal blood flow decreases. In the clinical evaluation of patients suspected to suffer from FLD or Pick's disease, the absence of frontal rCBF diminutions is thus a strong sign speaking against such a diagnosis. If bilateral frontal flow decreases are found, several other brain disorders have to be considered before suggesting a diagnosis of FLD or Pick's disease. Frontal flow pathology has been reported for instance in schizophrenia [12] and toxic encephalopathy due to abuse of alcohol [13] or long-term exposure to organic solvents [14].

rCBF achieves the best diagnostic value if serial recordings are made over several years. Such a case is illustrated in figure 1. Here the flow pathology is developing from a slight frontal disturbance to a very pronounced abnormality during clinical progress. We interpret these results as suggesting a progressive degenerative frontal lobe disorder of Pick or FLD type (autopsy is not yet available in this case).

Acknowledgement

Supported by the Swedish Medical Research Council (Project No. 4969).

References

1 Raichle ME, Grubb RL, Gado MH, Eichling JO, Ter-Pogossian MM: Correlation between regional cerebral blood flow and oxidative metabolism. Arch Neurol 1976;33:523–526.

2 Frackowiak RSJ, Pozzilli C, Legg NJ, Du Boulay GH, Marshall J, Lenzi GL, Jones T: Regional cerebral oxygen supply and utilization in dementia: A clinical and physiological study with oxygen-15 and positron tomography. Brain 1981;104:753–778.

3 Obrist WD, Thompson HK, Wang HS, Wilkinson WE: Regional cerebral blood flow estimated by 133-xenon inhalation. Stroke 1975;6: 245–256.

4 Risberg J, Ali Z, Wilson EM, Wills EL, Halsey JH: Regional cerebral blood flow by 133-xenon inhalation. Preliminary evaluation of an initial slope index in patients with unstable flow compartments. Stroke 1975;6:142–148.

5 Risberg J: Regional cerebral blood flow measurement by 133 Xe inhalation: Methodology and applications in neuropsychology and psychiatry. Brain Lang 1980;9:9–34.

6 Risberg J: Frontal lobe degeneration of non-Alzheimer type. III. Regional cerebral blood flow. Arch Gerontol Geriatr 1987;6:225–233.

7 Warkentin S, Passant U, Brun A, Risberg J, Gustafson L: Cerebral blood flow in dementia related to neuropathological findings. Neurobiol Aging 1992;13(suppl 1):96.

8 Brun A: Frontal lobe degeneration of non-Alzheimer type. I. Neuropathology. Arch Gerontol Geriatr 1987;6:193–208.

9 Risberg J: Development of high-resolution two-dimensional measurement of regional cerebral blood flow; in Wade J, Knezevic S, Maximilian VA, Mubrin Z, Prohovnik I (eds): Impact of Functional Brain Imaging in Neurology and Psychiatry. London, John Libbey, 1987, pp 35–43.

10 Hagstadius S, Risberg J: Regional cerebral blood flow characteristics and variations with age in resting normal subjects. Brain Cogn 1989;10:28–43.

11 Brun A, Englund E: A white matter disorder in dementia of the Alzheimer type: A pathoanatomical study. Ann Neurol 1986;19:253–262.

12 Ingvar DH, Franzén G: Abnormalities of cerebral blood flow distribution in patients with chronic schizophrenia. Acta Psychiatr Scand 1974;50:425–462.

13 Berglund M, Hagstadius S, Risberg J, Johanson AM, Bliding Å, Mubrin Z: Normalization of regional cerebral blood flow in alcohols during the first 7 weeks of abstinence. Acta Psychiatr Scand 1987;75:202–208.

14 Risberg J, Hagstadius S: Effects of the regional cerebral blood flow of long-term exposure to organic solvents. Acta Psychiatr Scand 1983; 67(suppl 303):92–99.

Dementia 1993;4:188–191

Siegbert Warkentin
Ulla Passant

Department of Psychogeriatrics,
University Hospital, Lund, Sweden

Functional Activation of the Frontal Lobes

Regional Cerebral Blood Flow Findings in Normals and in Patients with Frontal Lobe Dementia Performing a Word Fluency Test

Key Words
Regional cerebral blood flow
Word fluency
Normals
Frontal lobe dementia

Abstract
The present study examined the utility of the Word Fluency Test (WFT) as a frontal-lobe-activating test in brain imaging. Regional cerebral blood flow (rCBF) was measured during rest and during the WFT in 49 healthy volunteers and in 15 patients with frontal lobe dementia (FLD). The results showed a highly significant frontal lobe activation in 85% of the normal subjects. This finding was not related to age or to the level of performance on the WFT. A significant frontal activation was seen in 13 of the 15 FLD patients. The frontal flow increase did not reach normal levels, and was not related to age, illness duration or severity of clinical symptoms. The results suggest that the WFT is an ideal test to use in conjunction with functional imaging in normals as well as in patients with organic dementia.

Much research in human neuropsychology has been devoted to the study of human prefrontal functions and the role of the prefrontal cortex in mental activity. The bulk of knowledge has been primarily obtained with brain-injured patients [1]. By means of brain imaging methods which provide a dynamic functional view of the brain, such as assessment of the regional cerebral blood flow (rCBF), it is possible to advance our knowledge of the cortical functional substrates of cognition [2, 3].

One of the more promising ways to study brain function is the use of activation paradigms, in which subjects are studied before and during performance of a cognitive task. In this way it is possible to evaluate the relationship between performance of a particular task and regional alterations in brain activity which are associated with that task [4]. An important aspect of this approach is that, once it is established that a certain task detectably and consistently activates particular brain regions in normals, one can extend the findings of such stimulation to the study of patients. In this way, an activation protocol may be useful in evaluating the functional capacity of the brain, by its use as a form of 'stress test'.

Fig. 1. Topographic group mean rCBF (32 detectors) in normals, showing the vertex view of the cerebral cortex with the frontal pole at the top and the left hemisphere to the left. The colors represent flow distribution values (f_1, regional values in percent of the global mean) as defined by the key to the far right. The activation response (Diff, shown at the bottom) was calculated by subtracting each detector value obtained during the task from the corresponding values at rest.

Fig. 5. Topographic group mean rCBF (254 detectors) in FLD patients. Note the activation response (Diff) in the lower frontal and frontotemporal areas in both hemispheres.

Siegbert Warkentin, PhD
CBF Laboratory
Department of Psychogeriatrics
University Hospital
S–221 85 Lund (Sweden)

1013–7424/93/0044–0188
$2.75/0

1

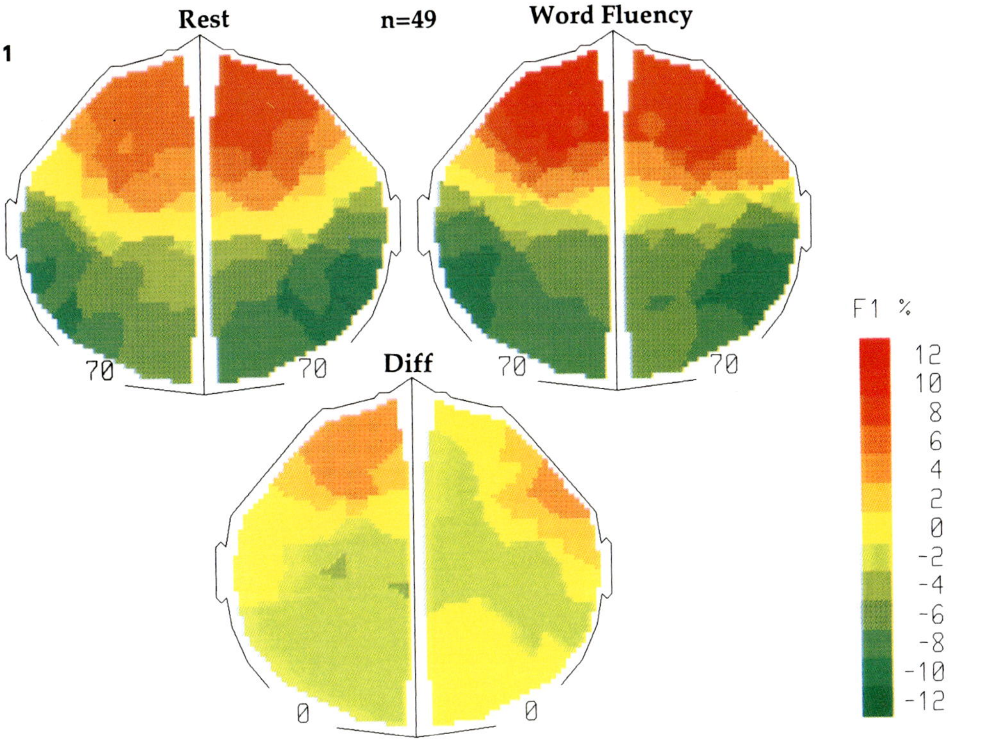
Rest
n=49
Word Fluency
70
70
70
70
Diff
0
0
F1 %
12
10
8
6
4
2
0
-2
-4
-6
-8
-10
-12

5

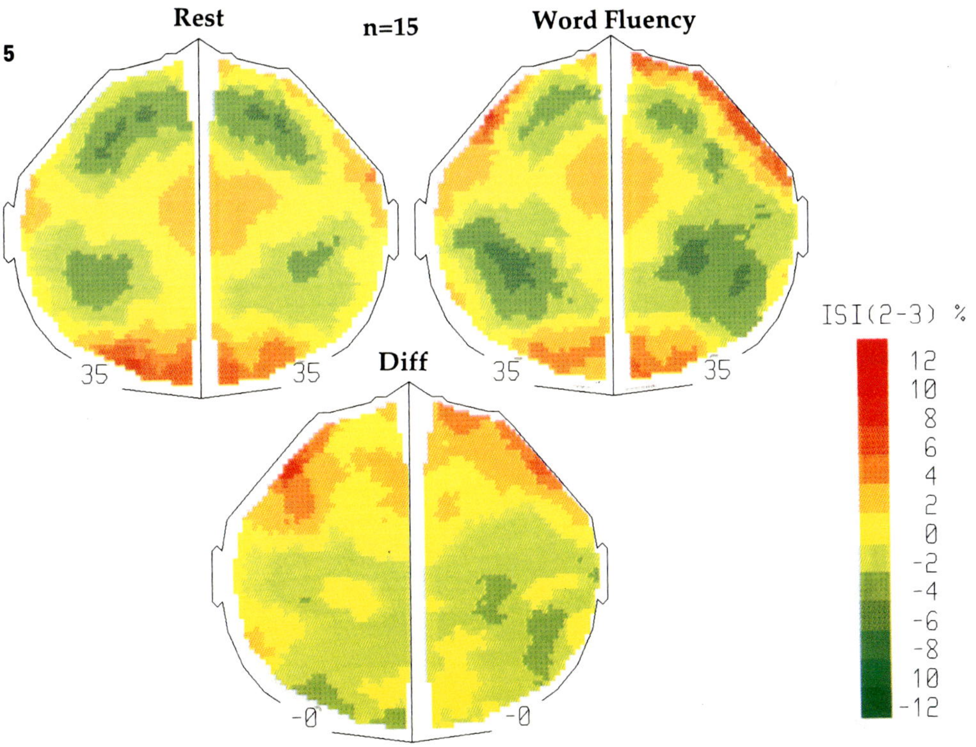
Rest
n=15
Word Fluency
35
35
35
35
Diff
-0
-0
ISI(2-3) %
12
10
8
6
4
2
0
-2
-4
-6
-8
10
-12

Previous research on brain-injured patients has found that the Word Fluency Test (WFT) is sensitive to the presence of frontal lobe lesions [5]. This task is ideal to use in conjunction with functional imaging in that it is simple to perform and maintains the subject in a relatively constant state of cognitive activity. However, few functional imaging studies have used the WFT in normal subjects [6–8] and the findings were based on small subject samples. If one is to use the WFT as a frontal stress test in activation paradigms, an important question is to investigate how reproducible and consistent the frontal activation is in relatively large samples of subjects. Therefore, the present investigation was conducted to: (1) test the reliability of the WFT as a frontal-lobe-activating test in normal subjects; (2) study the relationship between performance on WFT and functional cortical activation, and (3) investigate the utility of WFT as a stress test in patients with frontal lobe dementia.

Material and Methods

Subjects

The subjects comprised two groups: (1) 49 normal volunteers (29 males) who gave their informed consent. All were right handed and screened for the absence of psychiatric and somatic illness. Mean age of the group was 33 years (age range 21–62). (2) 15 patients (M/F 5/10) with frontal lobe dementia of non-Alzheimer type (FLD). Mean age was 62 years (age range 41–76) and mean duration of illness was 4.5 years (range 2–8). The diagnosis was based on neuropsychiatric and, neuropsychological evaluations, and on the findings obtained by CT, SPECT, EEG, and MRI.

Regional Cerebral Blood Flow

The rCBF was measured by the xenon-133 inhalation method developed by Obrist et al. [9] and modified by Risberg et al. [10]. The inert gamma-radiating tracer xenon-133 (90 MBq/l) was inhaled for 1 min through a face mask followed by 10 min of breathing of ordinary air. In the present study we used 32 scintillation detectors arranged in a radial array around the head (Inhalation Cerebrograph 32 C, Novo Diagnostic Systems, Hadsund Denmark) for the normal subjects. The FLD patients were measured by a high-resolution system with 254 probes (Cortexplorer 256 HR, Scan, Detectronics Inc., Hadsund, Denmark). The air passage artifact was corrected as suggested by Risberg [2].

Head position was kept constant by the use of four projection lights, which aligned the detector assembly with the auditory meatuses and the outer canthuses in a standardized manner. The arterial pCO_2 level was estimated from the expired end-tidal CO_2 values.

Procedure

The subjects underwent two rCBF measurements, one during rest and one during performance of the WFT [11]. The test was slightly modified in order to be suitable for the rCBF measurement. The subjects were instructed to say aloud as many words they could think of beginning with a specified target letter (e.g., F, A, S). Letters were changed at 1-min intervals and the responses were recorded on tape. The test score was the number of words produced per minute, excluding perseverations.

The measurement procedure was explained to the subjects before each study, and they were told to keep their eyes closed under the eye pads. The measurements were performed in the same order (rest, test) in all the subjects.

The task commenced 2 min prior to xenon inhalation and continued throughout the entire measurement period of 11 min.

The study was approved by the Lund University Ethical Committee and the Radiation Safety Committee.

Statistical Analysis

The raw values of each probe were used to compute the mean CBF values. Changes in CBF and rCBF (raw values in ml/100 g/min as well as distribution values in percent of hemispheric mean) from rest to test were analyzed by using the paired t test and Wilcoxon's matched pairs signed rank test.

Results

Normal Subjects

The mean rCBF distributions for the normal subjects during rest and during the WFT are illustrated in figure 1. Mean hemispheric blood flow did not change significantly from rest to test, but a significant difference between the hemispheres was seen during WFT, with higher values on the left side.

The typical hyperfrontal flow distribution was seen during both rest and during WFT, with relatively higher values in frontal areas and lower values in postcentral areas. The bottom illustration in figure 1 shows the difference in regional flow between the measurements obtained by subtracting the values at rest from those during WFT.

This subtraction thus represents the actual activation response, i.e. which areas showed increased blood flow during WFT. The results show a significant flow increase in the left anterior frontal and inferior frontal areas, together with a significant reduction of flow in the upper central and anterior parietal areas. In addition, right frontotemporal values were significantly higher during the WFT than during rest.

An analysis of the individual responses revealed that 41/49 subjects (85%) showed a flow increase in the left and/or right frontal areas. Of the 41 subjects with frontal activation, 35 (71%) showed a left over right increase, while the remaining 14 subjects showed no frontal increase or even a slight deactivation from rest to the WFT. These findings are illustrated in figures 2 and 3. In the group of so-called 'nonactivators', the values during rest in the left frontal areas were significantly higher than

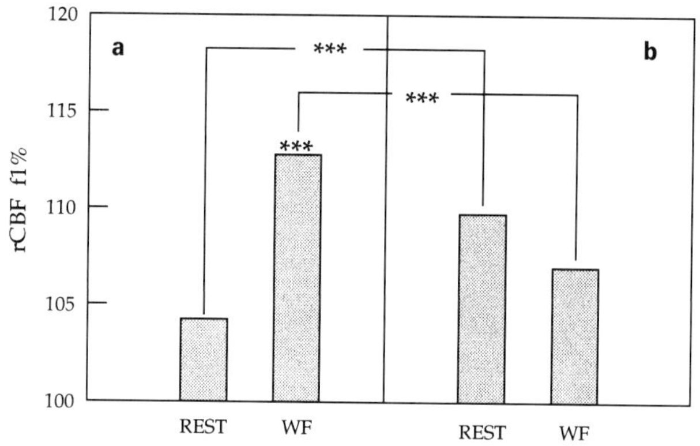

2

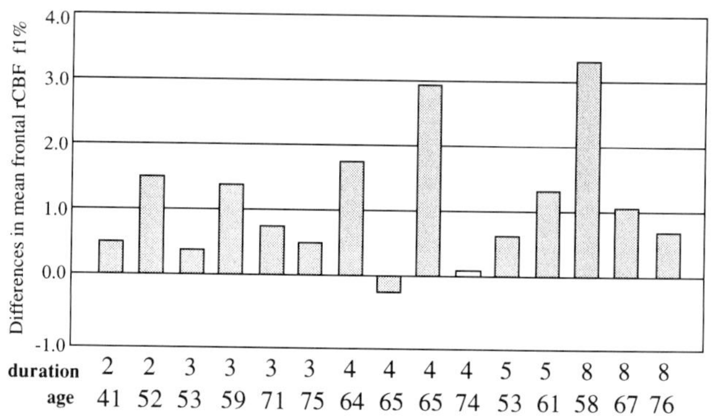

6

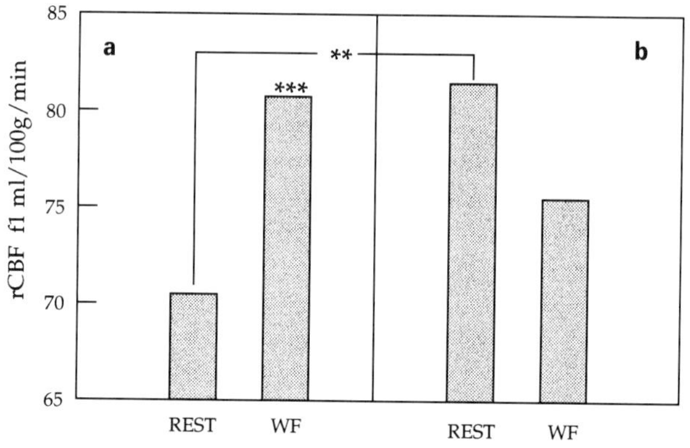

3

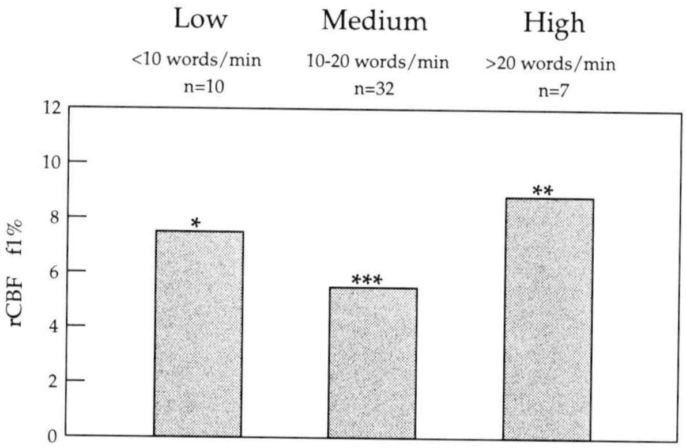

4

Fig. 2. Group mean values of superior frontal and frontotemporal areas of the left hemisphere in normal subjects. Bars represent f_1 distribution values (in percent of the global mean). Student's t test: *** $p < 0.001$. **a** Activators (n = 35). **b** Nonactivators (n = 14).

Fig. 3. Group mean values of superior frontal and frontotemporal areas of the left hemisphere in normal subjects. Bars represent actual flow values in ml/100 g/min. Student's t test: ** $p < 0.01$; *** $p < 0.001$. **a** Activators (n = 31). **b** Nonactivators (n = 18).

Fig. 4. Bars represent the activation response (distribution values, WFT – rest) in the left superior frontal and frontotemporal areas in normal subjects. Wilcoxon's signed rank test: * $p < 0.05$; ** $p < 0.01$; *** $p < 0.001$.

Fig. 6. The bars represent the individual activation response (WFT – rest) in the mean superior frontal and frontotemporal areas in 15 FLD patients. Although the activation did not reach normal values, it was very consistent and highly significant for the group (Wilcoxon's matched pairs signed rank test; $p < 0.001$).

those of the 'activators'. This indicates that in the minority of subjects in whom no additional flow augmentation was seen during word production, the flow increase during WFT may have been concealed by their already initially higher resting values.

In order to investigate whether the subject's skill (i.e. performance in words/min) was related to frontal lobe activation, we divided the total subject group into 'low', 'medium' and 'high' performers. The results, which are shown in figure 4, revealed significant and quite similar flow increases in all the groups, suggesting that the frontal flow increase was not related to the performance on the WFT.

Patients with FLD

Figure 5 shows the blood flow pattern in FLD patients. The mean hemispheric blood flow was significantly below normal values, during rest as well as during the WFT. The flow distribution showed the typical flow decrease in frontal areas bilaterally with relatively spared postcentral areas. During the WFT, however, a significant flow increase was seen in frontotemporal and superior frontal areas in both hemispheres. This frontal increase was seen in 13 of the 15 patients and thus a relatively consistent finding, as shown in figure 6. The activation response did, however, not reach the level of normals and the performance level was also clearly subnormal. There was no relation between the frontal activation response and age, duration of illness, or the clinical severity of the diseases.

Discussion

The findings have shown that the WFT activates the dorsolateral and frontotemporal cortex in most normal subjects, especially in the left hemisphere. Thus, the results suggest that the WFT is a reliable test to use in activation paradigms and to study the functional capacity of the frontal lobes with brain imaging. Our findings are also consistent with some PET studies which have shown increased metabolic rates in frontal areas during the WFT [6–8].

We found no correlation between performance on the WFT and rCBF. However, the subjects who showed a frontal elevation of rCBF from rest to the WFT had significantly lower frontal values during rest compared to those who showed no frontal increase. In a recent PET study a correlation was found between the relative metabolic rates of the frontal lobes and verbal fluency such that high performers had a lower resting metabolism than low performers [12]. These observations might reflect behavioral differences in the resting situation in which subjects who activate their frontal cortex have a relative economy of effort and cognitive efficiency during rest. For the subjects with more elevated baseline values, the resting state may have been characterized by an ongoing internal monologue and thus a true activation response may have been concealed.

Our findings also showed that the actual production of words or spoken language was not a critical factor for the frontal activation. This is consistent with the findings by Frith et al. [6] that the frontal activation is not modality specific but may be more generally associated with internal response generation by willed action.

In the group with FLD, bilateral frontal activation was seen in 13 of the 15 patients, primarily in the frontotemporal areas. Although these findings are very preliminary by the very nature of their uniqueness, they indicate that these patients do seem to have some spared functional capacity (maybe in terms of arousability) in their frontal lobes, even after many years of illness.

In conclusion, the results of the present study point to the usefulness of the WFT as a frontal-lobe-activating test in brain imaging. The relative ease with which this test can be administered makes it particularly suitable as a research instrument in patients who, by the very nature of their clinical condition, have a limited performance capacity.

Acknowledgements

Supported by the Swedish Medical Research Council (Project No. 4969).

Special thanks to eng. Siv Karlson for preparing the illustrations.

References

1 Milner B: Some effects of frontal lobotomy in man; in Warren JM, Akert K (eds): The frontal granular cortex and behavior. New York, McGraw-Hill, 1964, pp 313–334.

2 Risberg J: Regional cerebral blood flow measurements by 13-Xe inhalation. Methodology and applications in neuropsychology and psychiatry. Brain Lang 1980;6:225–233.

3 Ingvar DH: Serial aspects of language and speech related to prefrontal cortical activity. A selective review. Hum Neurobiol 1983;2:177–189.

4 Warkentin S, Risberg J, Nilsson A, Karlson S, Graae E: Cortical activity during speech production. A study of regional cerebral blood flow in normal subjects performing a word fluency task. Neuropsychiat Neuropsychol Beh Neurol 1991;4:305–316.

5 Crockett D, Bilsker D, Hurwitz T, Kozak J: Clinical utility of three measures of frontal lobe dysfunction in neuropsychiatric samples. Int J Neurosci 1986;30:241–248.

6 Frith CD, Friston K, Liddle PF, Frackowiak RSJ: Willed action and the prefrontal cortex in man: A study with PET. Proc R Soc Lond B 1991;244:241–246.

7 Frith CD, Friston KJ, Liddle PF, Frackowiak RSJ: A Pet study of word finding. Neuropsychologia 1991;12:1137–1148.

8 Parks RW, Loewenstein DA, Dodrill KL, Barker WW, Yoshii F, Chang JY, Emran A, Apicella A, Sheremata WA, Duara R: Cerebral metabolic effects of a verbal fluency test: A PET scan study. J Clin Exp Neuropsychol 1988;10:565–575.

9 Obrist WD, Thompson HK, Wang HS, Wilkinson WE: Regional cerebral blood flow estimated by 133-Xe inhalation. Stroke 1975;6: 245–256.

10 Risberg J, Ali Z, Wilson EM, Wills EL, Halsey JH: Regional cerebral blood flow by 133-Xe inhalation. Preliminary evaluation of an initial slope index in patients with unstable flow compartments. Stroke 1975;6:142–148.

11 Benton AL: Differential behavioral effects in frontal lobe disease. Neuropsychologia 1968;6: 53–60.

12 Boivin MJ, Giordani B, Berent S, Amato DA, Lehtinen S, Koeppe RA, Buchtel HA, Foster NL, Kuhl DE: Verbal fluency and positron emission tomographic mapping of regional cerebral glucose metabolism. Cortex 1992;28: 231–239.

Dementia 1993;4:192–203

Robert P. Friedland[a]
Elisabeth Koss[a]
Alan Lerner[a]
Peter Hedera[a]
William Ellis[c]
Nina Dronkers[d]
Beth A. Ober[d]
William J. Jagust[b]

[a] Alzheimer Center, University Hospitals of Cleveland, Ohio;
Departments of
[b] Neurology and
[c] Pathology, University of California, Davis, Calif.;
[d] Department of Applied Behavioral Sciences, University of California, Davis, Calif., USA

Functional Imaging, the Frontal Lobes, and Dementia

Key Words
Dementia
Frontal lobe dementia
Pick's disease
Positron emission tomography
Scopolamine
Echolalia

Abstract
A 58-year-old man developed progressive difficulty with comprehension and verbal output with dementia. Positron emission tomography with ^{18}F 2-fluoro-2-deoxy-*D*-glucose demonstrated asymmetrical frontal and anterior temporal lobe loss of glucose use. Scopolamine infusion (0.3 mg) did not influence memory. Postmortem studies revealed evidence of Pick's disease, with Pick bodies, loss of somatostatin, preservation of choline acetyltransferase and immunostaining with neurofilament antibodies. Pharmacological challenge and positron imaging offer valuable means for the noninvasive assessment of dementing illness. The contributions of functional imaging to our knowledge of frontal involvement in dementing illness are reviewed.

The neurodegenerations of the aging brain are a complex and interrelated set of illnesses. Alzheimer's disease (AD), Pick's disease, frontal lobe dementia (FLD), Parkinson's disease, progressive supranuclear palsy (PSP) and amyotrophic lateral sclerosis are all distinct entities which, on occasion, share important behavioral and pathological characteristics. We have known about Parkinson's disease since 1817, and about AD since 1906 – yet we are still puzzled by their common co-occurrence, as well as by the motor features of AD, and the cognitive features of Parkinson's disease. Our knowledge of these disorders is based largely upon studies obtained after death, at the 'end-stage' of disease processes. Functional imaging with positron emission tomography (PET) and single photon emission computed tomography (SPECT) provides us with quantitative measures of the brain's vital functions during life. In this paper we present an autopsy-confirmed case of Pick's disease studied with PET and with a psychopharmacological paradigm which revealed the relative integrity of central cholinergic systems in vivo. We review the use of PET in studies of Pick's disease and frontal lobe dementia. Alterations of frontal lobe function detected in AD in PET studies are also discussed.

Case Report

A 61-year-old left-handed retired aerospace engineer (R.M.) with onset of neurological dysfunction in 1979 was first seen at the Veterans Administration Medical Center, Martinez, Calif., in October 1982. He had a 3-year history of progressive difficulty in understanding what was said to him and repeating what he had been told, as well as increasing agitation. Past medical history, family history, social history and review of symptoms were not contributory. General

Preliminary accounts of this work have been presented [1, 2].

R.P. Friedland, MD
Alzheimer Center
University Hospital of Cleveland
2074 Abington Road
Cleveland, OH 44106 (USA)

medical and neurological exams were otherwise not remarkable and routine blood and urine tests were normal. He developed visual hallucinations in 1983. Bradykinesia, masked facies and echolalia was observed late in the illness which was rapidly progressive and he died in 1985.

Neuropsychological Testing

At the time of initial evaluation the patient was oriented with respect to place but not to time. He knew the year but not the month, date or day of the week. His initial Mattis Dementia Rating Scale [3] score was 100, indicating mild-to-moderate impairment. There was poor short-term and long-term memory and he was easily distracted. He performed above average on the block design subtest of the Wechsler Adult Intelligence Scale (WAIS) [4]. There was a 20-point difference between the verbal IQ and performance IQ scales of the WAIS. Digit span was relatively unaffected. His performance on these WAIS subtests were virtually the same 6 months later, but performance on the vocabulary subtest had declined from a scaled score of 6 to a scaled score of 2. By the third evaluation his echolalia had progressed to the point where administration of the verbal subtest was not possible. There was decline at that point on digit symbol and block design and the Mattis Dementia Rating Scale score declined to 78 at the third evaluation. Performance on tests of verbal fluency, verbal conceptualization, and verbal memory all declined from the initial exam, as did performance on visual conceptualization subtests [5]. He showed no difficulty in drawing or in spatial orientation tasks.

Language testing at the time of initial evaluation revealed speech which was well articulated, although aprosodic and with many grammatical errors, pause fillers and paraphasias. There was a marked deficit in auditory comprehension with agrammatic language production, though phrase length was normal. The patient did worse on tasks which involved manipulation of grammatical structures, such as auditory comprehension of commands and complex ideational material, repetition of sentences, reading sentences and paragraphs and writing. His scores on part A of the Token test were near normal, but his performance declined markedly on part F of the Token test which requires comprehension of more complex syntactic structure [6]. His comprehension and productive use of single words was relatively intact and he had trouble putting sentences together. Performance on language tasks involving syntactic manipulation was poor, as reflected by low and continuously declining scores on sentence comprehension and production. He subsequently developed progressive nonfluent aphasia with impaired verbal memory.

On initial exam auditory comprehension and repetition of single words, writing of automatic sequences and single words, recitation of automatic series, singing and rhythm was relatively intact, as was his oral reading. Subsequent exam revealed continued decline, particularly in oral and written expression and auditory comprehension. He eventually became mute and unresponsive in January 1985 after passing through a stage in which he repeated everything said to him. He was unresponsive even to automatized phrases during this time.

The patient's visual-spatial and performance skills were remarkably unimpaired and remained so over time. His initial performance on tasks such as selective reminding [7] was closer to that of normal elderly subjects than to that of Alzheimer patients. On the early tests the patient showed good performance on copying and other tasks from the Boston Parietal Lobe Battery [5]. Map performance was preserved. He was skilled in written calculations and performed nearly perfectly on tests of right-left orientation. Right-left orientation failed markedly by the 4th year of the illness. At the initial evaluation there was a marked learning deficit as revealed by the California Verbal Learning Test [8]. He was unable to recall any items from the list after a 20-min delay, even with category cues. On the Wechsler Memory Scale of logical memory only 99% of idea units were recalled [9]. Five (one half) of the total number of designs on the Benton Visual Retention test [10] were preserved. Follow-up testing showed steadily decreasing performance on selective reminding with poor performance on discourse memory and memory for designs. Performance on the Purdue Peg Board [11] was intact on the first two sessions (tables 1, 2).

Pharmacological Testing

In early 1983 a double-blind study of the effect of a muscarinic blocker was performed in order to assess the integrity of central cholinergic systems. Intravenous scopolamine infusion (0.3 mg) had no effect on verbal memory as measured by the Buschke Selective Reminding test [7]. This is in contrast to the marked effect of low dose scopolamine on memory in Alzheimer's disease patients [12, 13].

Laboratory Studies

Successive X-ray computed tomographic images show progressive extensive atrophy of the anterior temporal lobes, with lesser atrophy of the anterior and medial surfaces of the frontal lobes (fig. 1). There is also enlargement of the temporal horns of the lateral ventricles. The electroencephalograph was normal in 1982 and 1983. Brain stem auditory evoked potentials, middle latency auditory evoked potentials, somatosensory evoked potentials and pattern reversal visual evoked potential were all normal in 1982. PET with 18-fluorodeoxyglucose (FDG) using the Donner 280-crystal tomograph in January, 1983 (the 4th year of the illness) revealed marked bilateral anterior temporal and anterior frontal hypometabolism (fig. 1). There was also globally diminished metabolism, especially in right greater than left anterior temporal cortex and inferior frontal cortex (table 3).

Neuropathology and Neurochemistry

Gross examination revealed marked cerebral cortical atrophy with extremely widened sulci in the anterior temporal lobes bilaterally, and to a lesser degree, in the anterior frontal lobes. Microscopic examination showed many neurons in temporal cortex in hippocampus with cytoplasmic inclusions typical of Pick's cells. Many cells were vacuolated and fibrillary with some dense glossy inclusions. There were no neurons remaining in the maximally atrophic temporal cortex. The cortex was filled with numerous small fibrillary astrocytes with prominent eosinophilic processes. Lipofuscin was abundant in the astrocytes and in the intervening neuropil. In some regions deeper cortical laminae were replaced by a row of small cysts. Many surviving neurons in these maximally involved areas contained small amounts of cytoplasm filled with lipofuscin and a few contained cytoplasmic masses that were amphophilic or slightly basophilic and generally finely striated or vacuolated. Capillaries with thick PAS-positive walls were scattered throughout the degenerated cortex. The frontal cortex was well preserved in comparison to the temporal cortex and showed only mild gliosis and neuronal loss. Widely scattered neurons contained large amounts of glassy, slightly eosinophilic cytoplasm and many neurons were engorged with lipofuscin. Neurons were reasonably well preserved in the hippocampus but many contained large amounts of cytoplasm that was either

Table 1. Neuropsychological testing

Test	Normal or maximum score[a]	Oct 82	April 83	Nov 83	April 84
Mattis	max = 144	100	97	75	73
WAIS (scaled scores)					
Vocabulary	norm = 10	6	2	0	0
Digit-span	norm = 10	11	9	9	9
Digit symbol	norm = 10	9	11	9	8
Block design	norm = 10	13	12	10	na
Visuo-spatial Tasks					
Drawings					
command	max = 7	6	7	7	7
copy	max = 7	7	7	7	7
US map	max = 14	14	14	14	14
Calculations	max = 32	31	30	28	28
Right-Left	max = 16	13	13.50	7	na
Attention and speeded performance					
Trails A, s	norm = 48	27	25	na	na
Trails B, s	norm = 119	216	70	na	na
Letter canc	norm = na	26	37	33	32
Memory					
Selective reminding	norm = 75	58	42	31	na
CVLT	norm = 46	15	20	17	6
WMS Logical Memory	norm = 7.34	2	5	0	0
Benton Visual Retention	norm = 7[b]	5	5	4	na
Purdue Pegboard					
M single hand	norm = 17.37	14.25	13.75	na	na
M both hands	norm = 14.10	9	11	na	na

CVLT = California Verbal Learning Test.

[a] On tests for which a maximum score is given, normal subjects are expected to obtain that score. Each normal score was obtained for a standardization sample of elderly persons in an age range which included R.M.'s age (64). The normal scores for these various tests are presented in Lezak [98], except for letter cancellation, selective reminding, and the CVLT (see text for details).

[b] Norms for this test are available for different levels of premorbid IQ; the expected score here is 55- to 64-year-olds with a premorbid IQ above 110.

finely vacuolated or contained fine basophilic fibrils. Substantia nigra neurons were well preserved and there were no neural Lewy bodies or other characteristic inclusions within the substantia nigra or elsewhere. The neuronal inclusions were rarely homogeneous, as usually found in Pick's disease, but more often striated or finely vacuolated and rarely truly basophilic. There were no neuritic plaques or neurofibrillary tangles. Figure 2 shows Pick bodies from the temporal cortex stained with monoclonal antibody NP-16. There was also light to moderate staining of the Pick bodies with Sternberger's phosphorylated neurofilament antibody. Neurochemical studies of choline acetyltransferase and somatostatin are shown in table 2 (postmortem delay was 4 h). Elevated choline acetyltransferase activity was demonstrated with markedly reduced somatostatin content (table 4).

Table 2. Patient's raw score performance on subtests of the Boston Diagnostic Aphasia Examination and Token Test, measured at three 6-month intervals[1]

	Maximum possible score	Oct 82	May 83	Nov 83
Fluency[2]				
Articulation rating	7	7	6	6
Phrase-length rating	7	7	4	2
Verbal agility	14	14	14	10
Auditory Comprehension[2]				
Word discrimination	72	72	70.5	69
Body-part identification	20	NA	20	17
Commands	15	13	9	4
Complex ideational material	12	2	2	0
Naming[2]				
Responsive naming	30	12	10	0
Visual confrontation naming	105	91	87	79
Animal naming	23	9	8	7
Body part naming	30	29	30	22
Oral Reading[2]				
Word reading	30	30	30	27
Sentence reading	10	9	9	8
Repetition[2]				
Repetition of words	10	10	10	9
High probability sentences	8	3	3	3
Low probability sentences	8	2	2	0
Reading Comprehension[2]				
Symbol discrimination	10	10	10	9
Word recognition	8	NA	8	8
Comprehension of oral spelling	8	7	7	7
Word-picture matching	10	NA	9	10
Reading sentences & paragraphs	10	4	6	4
Writing[2]				
Mechanics	3	3	3	3
Serial writing	47	47	47	46
Primer-level dictation	15	15	15	15
Written confrontation naming	10	8	8	8
Spelling to dictation	10	8	10	9
Sentences to dictation	12	8	7	8
Narrative writing	4	3	2	1
Token Test				
A–E	67	66	66	67
F	96	80	62	53
Total	163	146	128	120

1 By 4/84 he was no longer testable.
2 Boston Diagnostic Aphasia Examination.

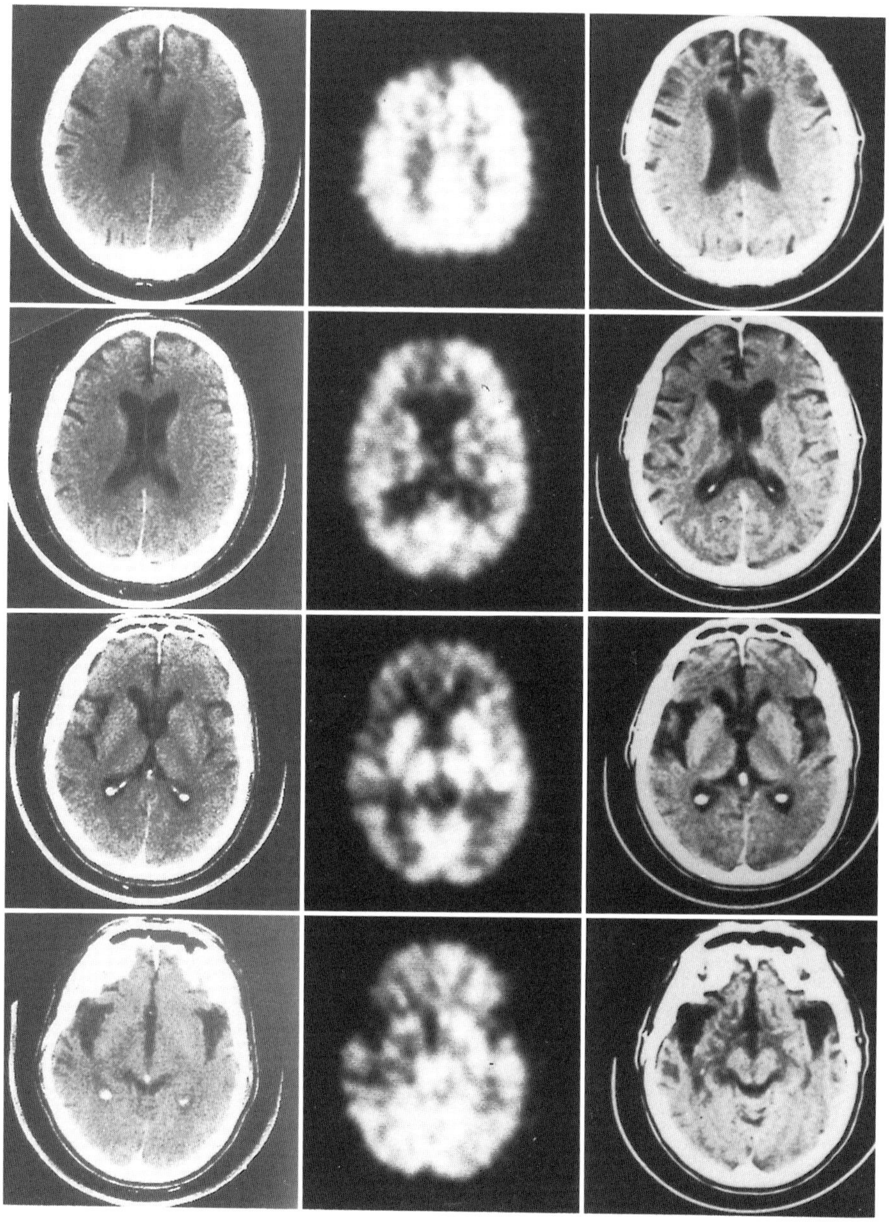

Fig. 1. Images from X-ray CT (12/82) left column, PET image of glucose utilization (1/83) center column, X-ray CT (4/84) right column. Note progressive severe cortical atrophy on CT images, most marked in frontal and anterior temporal cortices. PET images disclose marked anterior temporal and frontal hypometabolism, right worse than left. The patient's right side is presented on the left side of each of the images.

Discussion

This case demonstrates many interesting behavioral, neuropharmacological, neurochemical and pathological features. His language disturbance was unlike the language profile of Alzheimer patients, in which disturbances of lexical access and semantic processing are usually evident, with relative sparing of syntactic skills. Language dysfunction comparable to that observed in this case was noted by Arnold Pick in his original report [14]. Relative preservation of choline acetyltransferase activity has been found in other cases of Pick's disease together with depression of somatostatin content [15, 16]. This is in contrast to the diminished choline acetyltransferase content found in AD [17, 18]. These neurochemical findings are likely to be responsible for the lack of effect of cholinergic blockade upon memory functioning. Scopolamine challenge testing may provide a valuable noninvasive method for assessing central cholinergic integrity.

There have been few postmortem studies of Pick's disease cases assessed during life with PET. The observed pattern of diminished glucose use in anterior bitemporal

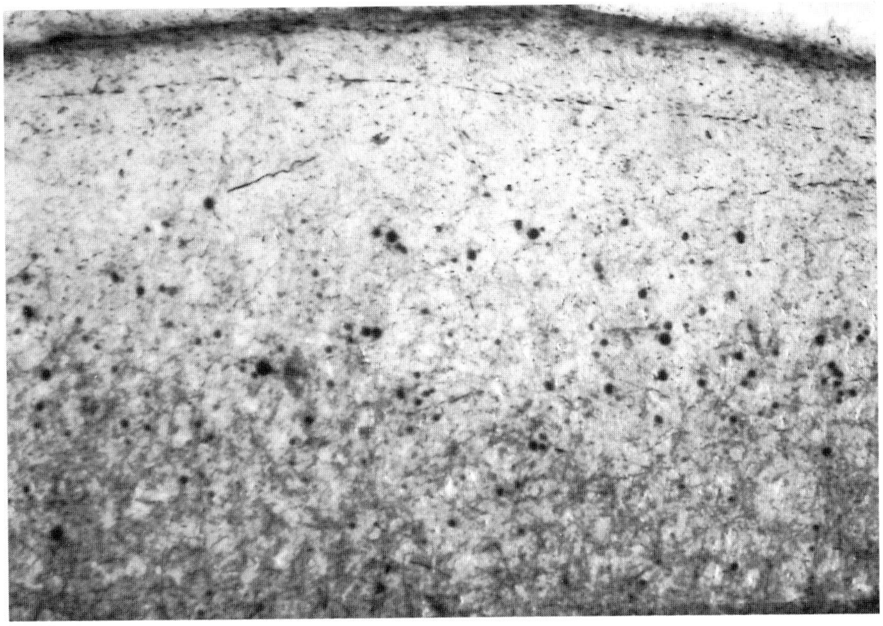

Fig. 2. NP 16 antibody immunostaining of cerebral cortex, disclosing ballooned neurons (courtesy of P. Davies, Albert Einstein College of Medicine, N.Y.).

Table 3. Rates of glucose utilization (mg/100 g/min) in case R.M. and in healthy aged controls (n = 7, mean age 63 years, SD 3.0, mean ± SD)

		Basal ganglia level		Mid ventricular level	
		Pick's	controls	Pick's	controls
Frontal cortex	L	4.48	6.23 ± 0.78	4.99	6.21 ± 0.81
	R	4.24	6.34 ± 0.81	4.34	6.51 ± 0.83
Temporal cortex	L	5.32	5.92 ± 0.77	–	–
	R	4.92	6.20 ± 0.64	–	–
Parietal cortex	L	–	–	5.82	6.17 ± 0.82
	R	–	–	5.00	6.64 ± 0.88
Entire cortex	L	4.93	6.00 ± 0.74	5.62	6.27 ± 0.84
	R	4.49	6.33 ± 0.70	5.05	6.63 ± 0.81

Table 4. Neurochemistry

	Choline acetyltransferase activity, Nm Ach produced/h/100 mg prot	Somatostatin concentration, ng/mg prot
This case	1,402	0.43
Healthy aged	306 ± 45	2.82 ± 0.45

Assay of frozen specimen taken from right anterior temporal cortex. Postmortem delay was 4 h. (Performed in the laboratory of Peter Davies, PhD, Albert Einstein College of Medicine, N.Y.)

cortex is markedly different from the bilateral posterior temporal-parietal hypometabolism seen in patients with Alzheimer's disease [19]. Temporal lobe accentuation of pathology in this case in reminiscent of that first reported by Malamud and Boyd [20], who point out that cases of Pick's disease with outstanding atrophy of the temporal lobe often present with aphasia. Aphasia was recognized as a feature of the disease in the original report by Pick in 1892. The asymmetry noted in the present case has not been often described in Pick's disease. Pick's original cases involved symmetrical atrophy [14].

The exact nature of Pick bodies is not clear but several studies have reported similarities between neuronal inclusions in Pick's disease and neurofibrillary tangles in AD [21]. Gambetti et al. [22] used polyclonal neurofilament antibodies and Munoz-Garcia and Ludwin [23] used monoclonal neurofilament antibodies to immunolabel Pick bodies. Paired helical filament antigens in Pick's disease have also been reported by Rasool and Selkoe [24].

PET and SPECT Studies of the Frontal Lobe in AD and Pick's Disease

Frontal lobe impairment has been associated with denial of illness in patients with AD [25]. Denial or unawareness of impairment in AD is known to be associated with confabulation, reduplicative delusions and disorientation, but it is not associated with severity of illness, or with disease duration. Resting regional cerebral glucose metabolism in 16 AD patients without denial/unawareness has been compared to 18 AD patients with denial/unawareness. Patients with denial/unawareness had lower glucose use in right ($p < 0.01$) and left ($p < 0.05$) prefrontal and right premotor cortices ($p < 0.01$) when compared to patients without denial/unawareness. Principal components analysis showed that the denial/unawareness group had relatively fewer patients belonging to the parietal temporal hypometabolism group which is dominant in AD. These data support the view that denial of illness is a reflection of frontal cortex impairment in AD [26]. Anosognosia has also been found to be related to frontal lobe dysfunction in AD as measured by psychological tests [27].

Our case with pathologically confirmed Pick's disease demonstrated marked reduction of frontal and anterior temporal cortical metabolism measured as FDG uptake with PET. Similar patterns of hypometabolism in Pick's disease have been reported in other cases with pathologically confirmed diagnoses studied by PET [28, 29] or with clinical diagnosis only [30, 31]. This is consistent with the distribution of cortical atrophy in Pick's disease [32]. Patients reported by Szelies and Karenberg had significantly reduced metabolism in the caudate nucleus and the case reported by Kamo had also signs of thalamic involvement [28, 31]. Basal ganglia hypometabolism may be caused by loss of activity in the frontal association cortex, which massively projects to caudate and thalamus [33].

Similar results of dominant frontal hypoperfusion and relative sparing of other parts of the brain have been reported with SPECT studies of rCBF in Pick's disease [34, 35]. The same flow pattern was also observed in one patient with only mild cortical frontal atrophy on CT examination described by Deisenhammer and coworkers. This supports the view that very low metabolic rates observed in Pick's disease reflects metabolic disturbances and not only partial volume effect due to marked atrophy [36].

Language disorder can be a prominent feature of Pick's disease [37]. One of the patients described by Salmon and Franck [29] presented with the syndrome of progressive aphasia and only later developed global deficit. The first PET examination in that case revealed reduction of FDG uptake limited to the left perisylvian area, and repeated examination after development of severe dementia also showed a bifrontal reduction. Study of patients with primary progressive aphasia without dementia have found similar patterns of pathology in perisylvian cortex of the dominant hemisphere, resembling the first examination in Salmon's and Franck's report [38, 39]. Our left-handed patient also had a remarkable language deficit in both expression and comprehension abilities and metabolic depression was higher in right frontal and anterior temporal areas. Correlation of language impairment and reduction of FDG uptake in Broca's area was also reported by Szelies and Karenberg [31].

The most characteristic finding in patients with AD using PET is a reduction of metabolism in postcentral parietal and temporal association cortex, which has been repeatedly confirmed in all stages of dementia [40–43]. These reports also stressed relative sparing of the frontal lobes compared to parietotemporal areas. Involvement of other parts of the brain remains more controversial. Considerable heterogeneity of PET findings in AD was stressed by Benson et al. [44], who found two different patterns of metabolic depression measuring FDG uptake: some patients had maximal hypometabolism in parietotemporal areas, while others had focal defects in frontal areas. Frackowiak et al. [45] measured utilization of $^{15}O_2$ in dementia of various etiologies. Depression of regional cerebral oxygen utilization ($rCMRO_2$) in frontal lobes was found in the subgroup of severely demented patients with degenerative dementia. During follow-up of 10 subjects with AD, 2 progressed from moderate to severe dementia, which was also associated with marked decline of global $CMRO_2$ and $rCMRO_2$ in premotor areas; this drop of prefrontal metabolism was out of proportion to parietal and temporal lobe decline. Reduction of absolute values of regional cerebral metabolic rate for glucose (rCMRglc) in the frontal lobe in severely demented patients has also been reported by others [46–48]. Jagust et al. [49] longitudinally followed 6 patients with AD; only the most severely demented patient in the study demonstrated significant decrease of frontal metabolism with the progression of the dementia.

McGeer et al. [50] found that the most significant frontal hypometabolism in AD was present in the group of severely demented patients. However, among their cases with clinical diagnoses of probable AD they also reported two moderately demented patients with isolated decline of frontal uptake of FDG; and 2 mildly impaired patients manifested reductions in the frontal area, but this was associated with marked reduction in parietal or temporal lobes as well. Depression of FDG uptake in frontal lobes in moderate dementia of the Alzheimer type has also been reported by Duara et al. [47], who found lower levels in left midfrontal gyrus in addition to parietal and temporal lobes. Prefrontal cortical areas had signs of hypometabolism of intermediate degree and orbitofrontal cortex demonstrated relative sparing along with primary sensomotor cortex [51]. Dynamic PET studies of glucose transport in AD revealed evidence for abnormality of forward glucose transport (significant reduction of K1*) in frontal and temporal lobes, which was also associated with decline of FDG uptake in the same areas [52].

Metabolic rates in middle frontal cortex negatively correlates with age in some studies of healthy aging, in contrast to temporal and parietal lobes [53–55]. The possible influence of age on frontal hypometabolism has also been analyzed in presenile (onset before age 65 years) and senile onset of AD [55]. Patients with earlier onset of dementia had focal metabolic disturbances, including also frontal lobes, and older patients demonstrated global reduction of FDG uptake without frontal involvement [55]: Koss et al. [56] found greater reduction of FDG uptake in the right hemisphere in younger patients with dominant asymmetry in the parietotemporal lobes. In contrast, older patients had more reduced metabolism in the left hemisphere, which included also significant frontal asymmetry and FDG uptake decline in left frontal cortex [56]. However, these differences between presenile and senile onset of AD and changing patterns of hypometabolism have not been confirmed by other authors, who have stressed parietal metabolic depression in both young and old AD groups [43, 57].

Resting neocortical rCMRglc patterns in AD have demonstrated left-right asymmetries which can be detected in early stages of dementia. Asymmetries in parietotemporal regions which do not favor either hemisphere with relative sparing of frontal regions have been reported [19]. Longitudinal studies have confirmed relative preservation of this asymmetry pattern in all but one patient [49]. Asymmetries in frontal associative cortex in the earliest stages of AD have also been reported [47, 58–62]. Left-right asymmetry often precedes clinical manifestation of AD [59]. Impaired function of frontal lobes and its projections was also supported by presence of crossed cerebellar diaschisis and uncrossed basal ganglia diaschisis in AD patients [63].

The study of the heterogeneity of the findings in AD has led to observations of correlations among psychometric functions and patterns of cortical metabolism. Among the right-handed patients with AD analyzed by Foster's group [64], disproportionate impairment of language functions was associated with decline of FDG uptake in left frontal areas, and metabolic activity in left frontal and parietal areas was correlated with verbal abilities. Haxby and Rapoport [65] compared left-right asymmetry of metabolism in association cortex with neuropsychological discrepancies between language and visuospatial skills using syntax/drawing index and index of performance on WAIS in tests of verbal arithmetic and immediate verbal memory (WAIS PDQ-MSQ). Syntax/drawing index correlated with cerebral metabolic asymmetries in frontal lobes (together with parietal) in the moderate AD patients, but not in mildly demented subjects. WAIS PDQ-MDQ correlated with asymmetries in frontal, temporal and parietal lobes, also in the moderate dementia subgroup [51, 65]. Disproportionate impairment of language functions was associated with lower left hemisphere rCMRglc, and more prominent visuospatial dysfunction with lower right hemisphere rCMRglc [65].

Performance on the WAIS has been correlated with metabolic activity in AD and healthy control subjects. Only one subtest was closely related to frontal cortex FDG uptake – the digit span subtest [41]. Association of impaired attention with frontal lobe hypometabolism has also been found in other studies [51, 66, 67]. Increased latencies of the P300 component of the event-related potential, reflecting perceptual recognition time, correlated with hypometabolism in parietal and frontal lobes in AD [68]. Analysis within the demented subjects found negative correlation of relative frontal hypometabolism and latency of P300, which is in agreement with reports of relation of Digit Span Test and P300 latency [68, 69].

Chase et al. [42] described one patient with AD with prominent frontal hypometabolism, who demonstrated significant attentional deficit together with personality changes. Correlation of disinhibition symptoms with reduction of frontal metabolism has been found in study of 3 AD patients with frontal lobe behavioral symptomatology: they had reductions of FDG uptake in prefrontal, orbitofrontal and anterior cingulate regions compared to controls and AD patients without behavioral disturbances [70]. Patients with behavioral symptomatology did not manifest more profound cognitive deficit than other AD subjects, which indicates a key role of frontal cortex pathology for behavioral symptoms, but not for cognitive decline [70].

Studies of cerebral blood flow, based on the coupling of brain metabolism and blood flow, have revealed ambiguous flow patterns in frontal regions. Analysis of 9 patients with AD with various severity of dementia, using SPECT with iofetamine ^{123}I (IMP) found a perfusion deficit in temporoparietal lobes with relative sparing of frontal lobes [71]. Hypoperfusion in frontal lobes (together with temporoparietal areas) measured by IMP SPECT has been suggested by Johnson et al. [72]. All patients in this study were severely demented in contrast to AD subjects reported by Jagust et al. [71]. These findings again point to decline of frontal lobe cerebral blood flow (CBF) with worsening of cognitive deficit, similarly to the results of PET studies [45, 47]. Relative decrease of CBF in frontal lobes with progression of dementia have also been reported by other authors [73, 74]. Correlation between severity of dementia and CBF was studied in 37 patients with AD and with different severity of dementia [75]. Decline in frontal lobes with progression of cognitive deficit was also noted in this study. Jagust et al. [76] found that younger patients had lower relative rCBF in left front lobes than older AD patients. Similar results suggesting correlation of language abilities and CBF in left frontal lobe has been reported by Burns et al. [77], who measured rCBF using ^{99m}Tc hexamethyl-propylenamine oxime (HMPAO). Burns et al. also found a negative relation between left frontal lobe CBF and the Mini-Mental State Examination (MMSE) score.

PET, SPECT and CBF Studies in Frontal Lobe Dementia

FLD is a form of primary degenerative dementia described by several groups in recent years [78–81]. The clinical picture is dominated by a ‘frontal lobe syndrome’ with changes in personality and behavior which are more prominent than memory or visual-spatial difficulties. Late in the course, a more generalized dementia may result. Some patients with FLD develop clinical signs of motor neuron disease [82, 83], which has also been called the amyotrophy dementia complex. Although FLD may comprise 10–15% of patients with dementia in some series [81, 84], relatively limited information regarding functional neuroimaging is available. This is partly due to difficulty in clinical diagnosis. Patients with FLD may fulfill DSM III-R [85] or NINCDS/ADRDA criteria [86] for probable Alzheimer disease. Pick’s disease may also present with prominent behavior change and FLD may represent some cases of ‘atypical Pick’s disease’ [84]. Pick’s disease presenting as motor neuron disease has also been described [87].

The rCBF findings in FLD have been consistent using a variety of techniques. Risberg [88] studied 9 FLD patients using ^{133}Xe inhalation to measure rCBF. He found reduced symmetric bifrontal blood flow, with preserved posterior cerebral blood flow. Follow-up of 7 patients over 2 years showed progression of the frontal flow deficit, but preservation of the overall rCBF pattern. Using HMPAO, Neary et al. [89] showed decreased frontal lobe metabolism in FLD and PSP. The two conditions often could be differentiated based on a preserved ‘rim’ of frontal cortical flow in PSP, using raters blinded to the clinical details. Miller et al. [90] studied FLD and AD using ^{133}Xe and HMPAO SPECT. Patients with FLD showed flow reductions in basal medial and dorsolateral frontal, and anterior temporal regions. Using the^{133}Xe inhalation technique, there was no overlap of FLD patients with normal age-matched controls in these areas. Smaller reductions were found in posterior parietal and posterior temporal regions. Patients with FLD and MND also showed bifrontal flow reductions using SPECT with ^{133}I-IMP [73].

Performance on clinical neuropsychological testing has paralleled the SPECT findings. Performance on the MMSE [91] was correlated with posterior parietal but not frontal rCBF in a group of FLD and AD patients [90]. However, other studies found significant correlations of MMSE performance with inferior frontal and parietal cortical CBF in FLD [92]. Impaired executive functioning correlating with hypoperfusion in dorsolateral frontal cortex has also been reported [90]. Elfgren et al. [93] reported a positive correlation between verbal ability and frontotemporal and superior frontal flow; spatial memory and visual-spatial ability correlated with temporal-parietal flow.

There is limited information available on the PET findings in FLD. Some of the patients of Chase et al. [94] may have had FLD. A recent study [95] found decreased rCBF and $CMRO_2$ in the frontal lobe exclusive of the precentral area in FLD as compared to AD. The reverse situation was found in parietal and occipital areas. Two patients with advanced FLD showed temporal reductions in rCBF and $rCMRO_2$. These findings are consistent with the more extensive data obtained from SPECT studies.

Prospects

Functional imaging has helped to define the metabolic and cerebrovascular concomitants of brain dysfunction in Pick's disease, AD and FLD. Regional CBF, PET and SPECT studies may assist in the evaluation of the differential diagnosis of dementing illnesses. Recent studies have demonstrated the potential for other imaging paradigms in application to the important clinical and research issues of AD and related disorders. Magnetic resonance imaging methods using fast sequences for the assessment of perfusion in brain have been reported [96]. It is hoped that the exquisite spatial and temporal resolution of magnetic imaging can be fruitfully applied to important issues of etiology, diagnosis and treatment of the neurodegenerative diseases of aging. Also, radiolabeled monoclonal antibodies targeting the Alzheimer amyloid beta protein have been developed for studies of cerebral amyloid angiopathy [97]. The development of a method for in vivo immunochemistry with neuroimaging will be a valuable adjunct to our current investigative techniques. We still have limited understanding of the vast clinical and biological heterogeneity of these illnesses. Integrative studies of brain physiology, genetics and epidemiology will be required to unravel these important questions.

Acknowledgements

The authors are indebted to P. Davies, PhD for neurochemical studies and to J. Borcich for neuropathological assistance.

Supported in part by the National Institutes of Health, Bethesda, Maryland (AG 08012-05) and by Philip Morris, USA.

References

1 Dronkers NS, Ober BA, Simpson GV, Friedland RP: Neuropsychological and physioanatomical features of suspected Pick's disease. Int Neuropsychol Soc Bull, 1984, p 13.
2 Friedland RP, Jagust WJ, Ober BA, Dronkers NF, Koss E, Simpson GV, Ellis WG, Budinger TF: The pathophysiology of Pick's disease. A comprehensive case study. Neurology 1986; 36(suppl 1):268.
3 Mattis S: Dementia Rating Scale Professional Manual. Odessa, Psychological Assessment Resources, 1988.
4 Wechsler DA: Wechsler Adult Intelligence Scale. Manual. New York, Psychological Corporation, 1955.
5 Goodglass H, Kaplan E: The Assessment of Aphasia and Related Disorders, ed 2. Philadelphia, Lea & Febiger, 1983.
6 De Renzi E, Vignolo LA: The Token Test: A sensitive test to detect disturbances in aphasics. Brain 1962;82:665–678.
7 Buschke H, Fuld PA: Evaluating storage, retention, and retrieval in disordered memory and learning. Neurology 1974;11:1019–1025.
8 Delis DC, Kramer JH, Kaplan E, Ober BA: The California verbal learning test-research edition. New York, The Psychological Corporation, 1987.
9 Wechsler DA: A standardized memory scale for clinical use. J Psychol 1945;19:87–95.
10 Benton Al: The Revised Visual Retention Test, ed 4. New York, Psychological Corporation, 1974.
11 Purdue Research Foundation: Examiner's Manual for the Purdue Pegboard. Chicago, Science Research Associates, 1948.
12 Sunderland T, Tariot PN, Mueller EA, Murphy DL, Weingardner H, Cohen RM: Cognitive and behavioral sensitivity to scopolamine in Alzheimer patients and controls. Psychopharmacol Bull 1985;21:676–679.
13 Sunderland T, Tariot PN, Weingartner H, Murphy DL, Newhouse PA, Mueller EA, Cohen RM: Pharmacological modelling of Alzheimer's disease. Prog Neuropsychopharmacol Biol Psychiatry 1986;10:599–610.
14 Pick A: Über die Beziehungen der senilen Hirnatrophie zur Aphasie. Prag Med Wochenschr 1892;17:165–172.
15 Yates CM, Simpson J, Maloney AFJ, Gordon A: Neurochemical observations in a case of Pick's disease. J Neurol Sci 1980;48:257–263.
16 Hansen LA, Deteresa R, Tobias H, Alford M, Terry RD: Cortical morphometry and cholinergic neurochemistry in Pick's disease. Am J Pathol 1988;131:507–518.
17 Whitehouse PJ, Price DL, Struble RG, Clark AW, Coyle JT, DeLong MR: Alzheimer's disease and senile dementia. Loss of neurons in the basal forebrain. Science 1982;215:1237–1239.
18 Wood PL, Hentienne P, Lal S, Nair NPV, Finlayson MH, Gauthier S, Palo J, Haltia M, Paetau A, Bird ED: A postmortem comparison of the cortical cholinergic system in Alzheimer's disease and Pick's disease. J Neurol Sci 1983; 62:211–217.
19 Friedland RP, Budinger TF, Koss E, Ober BA: Alzheimer's disease. Anterior-posterior and lateral hemispheric alterations in cortical glucose utilization. Neurosci Lett 1985;53:235–240.
20 Malamud N, Boyd DA Jr: Pick's disease with atrophy of the temporal lobes. Arch Neurol Psychiatry 1940;43:212–222.
21 Ulrich J, Haugh M, Anderton BH, Probst A, Lautenschlager C, His B: Alzheimer dementia and Pick's disease: Neurofibrillary tangles and Pick bodies are associated with identical phosphorylated neurofilament epitopes. Acta Neuropathol 1987;73:240–246.

22 Gambetti P, Shecket G, Getti B, et al: Neurofibrillary changes in human brain. An immunocytochemical study with a neurofillament antiserum. J Neuropathol Exp Neurol 1983;42:69–79.
23 Munoz-Garcia D, Ludwin SK: Classic and generalized variants of Pick's disease. A clinicopathological, ultrastructural, and immunocytochemical comparative study. Ann Neurol 1984;16:467–480.
24 Rasool CG, Selkoe DJ: Sharing a specific antigen by degenerating neurons in Pick's disease and Alzheimer's disease. N Engl J Med 1985; 312:700–705.
25 Nolan BH, Swihart AA, Pirozzolo FJ: The neuropsychology of normal aging and dementia. An introduction; in Wedding AM, Horton AM Jr, Webster J (eds): The Neuropsychology Handbook, New York, Springer, 1986, pp 410–440.
26 Friedland RP, Weinstein EA, Grady CL: Denial of illness is related to diminished frontal cortex glucose metabolism in Alzheimer's disease. Soc Neurosci Abstr 1992;18:735.
27 Michon A, Deweer B, Pillon B, Agid Y, Dubois B: Anosognia in SDAT is related to frontal lobe dysfunction. Neurology 1991;42:221.
28 Kamo H, McGeer PL, Herrop R, McGeer EG, Calne DB, Martin WRW, Pate DB: Positron emission tomography and histopathology in Pick's disease. Neurology 1987;37:439–445.
29 Salmon E, Franck G: Positron emission tomographic study in Alzheimer's disease and Pick's disease. Arch Gerontol Geriatr 1989 (suppl 1): 241–247.
30 Salmon E, Sadzot B, Franck G: Interest of positron emission tomography in the diagnosis of Pick's disease; in Bes et al. (eds): Senile Dementias: Early Detection. London, Libbey, 1986, pp 493–497.
31 Szelies B, Karenberg A: Störungen des Glukosestoffwechsels bei Pickscher Erkrankung. Fortschr Neurol Psychiatr 1986;54:393–397.
32 Knopman DS, Christensen KJ, Schut LJ, Harbaugh RE, Reeder T, Ngo T, Frey W II: The spectrum of imaging and neuropsychological findings in Pick's disease. Neurology 1989;39: 362–368.
33 Alexander GE, DeLong MD, Strick PL: Parallel organization of functionally segregated circuits linking basal ganglia and cortex. Annu Rev Neurosci 1986;9:357–381.
34 Deisenhammer E, Reisecker F, Leblhuber F, Holl K, Markut H, Trenkler J, Schneider I: Single-Photon-Emissions-Computertomographie bei der Differentialdiagnose der Demenz. Dtsch Med Wochenschr 1989;114:1639–1644.
35 Bonte FJ, Hom J, Tintner R, Weiner MF: Single photon tomography in Alzheimer's disease and the dementias. Semin Nucl Med 1990;20: 342–352.
36 Chawluk JB, Alavi A, Dann R, Hurtig HI, Bais S, Kushner MJ, Zimmerman RA, Reivich M: Positron emission tomography in aging and dementia. Effect of cerebral atrophy. J Nucl Med 1987;28:431–437.
37 Wechsler AF, Verity M, Rosenschein S, Fried I, Scheibel AB: Pick's disease. Arch Neurol 1982;39:287–290.
38 Gordon B, Selnes O: Progressive aphasia 'without dementia'. Evidence of more widespread involvement. Neurology 1984;34(suppl 1): 102.
39 Chawluk JB, Mesulam M-M, Hurtig H, Kushner M, Weintraub S, Saykin A, Rubin N, Alavi A, Reivich M: Slowly progressive aphasia without generalized dementia. Studies with positron emission tomography. Ann Neurol 1986; 19:68–74.
40 Friedland RP, Budinger TF, Ganz E, Yano Y, Mathis CA, Koss B, Ober BA, Huesman RH, Derenzo SE: Regional cerebral metabolic alterations in dementia of Alzheimer type. Positron emission tomography with [^{18}F]fluorodeoxyglucose. J Comput Assist Tomogr 1983;7:590–598.
41 Foster NL, Chase TN, Mansi L, Brooks R, Fedio P, Patronas NJ, di Chiro G: Cortical abnormalities in Alzheimer's disease. Ann Neurol 1984;16:649–654.
42 Chase TN, Foster NL, Fedio P, Brooks R, Mansi L, di Chiro G: Regional cortical dysfunction in Alzheimer's disease as determined by positron emission tomography. Ann Neurol 1984;15(suppl):S170–S174.
43 Small GW, Kuhl DE, Riege WH, Fujikawa DG, Ashford JW, Metter JE, Mazziotta JC: Cerebral glucose metabolic patterns in Alzheimer's disease. Effect of gender and age at dementia onset. Arch Gen Psychiatry 1989;46: 527–532.
44 Benson DF, Kuhl DE, Hawkins RA, Phelps ME, Cummings JL, Tsai SY: The fluorodeoxyglucose ^{18}F scan in Alzheimer's disease and multi-infarct dementia. Arch Neurol 1983;40: 711–714.
45 Frackowiak RSJ, Pozzilli C, Legg NJ, du Boulay GH, Marshall J, Lenzi GL, Jones T: Regional cerebral oxygen supply and utilization in dementia. A clinical and physiological study with oxygen-15 and positron tomography. Brain 1981;104:753–778.
46 de Leon MJ, Ferris SH, George AE, Christman DR, Fowler JS, Gentes C, Reisberg B, Gee B, Emmerich M, Yonekura Y, Brodie J, Kricheff II, Wolf A: Positron emission tomographic studies of aging and Alzheimer disease. AJNR 1983;4:568–571.
47 Duara R, Grady C, Haxby J, Sundaram M, Cutler NR, Heston L, Moore A, Schlageter N, Larson S, Rapoport SI: Positron emission tomography in Alzheimer's disease. Neurology 1986;36:879–887.
48 Fukuyama H, Harada K, Yamauchi H, Miyoshi T, Yamaguchi S, Kimura J, Kameyama M, Senda M, Yonekura Y, Konishi J: Coronal reconstruction images of glucose metabolism in Alzheimer's disease. J Neurol Sci 1991;106: 128–134.
49 Jagust WJ, Friedland RP, Budinger TF, Koss E, Ober B: Longitudinal studies of regional cerebral metabolism in Alzheimer's disease. Neurology 1988;38:909–912.
50 McGeer PL, Kamo H, Harrop R, Li DKB, Toukko H, McGeer EG, Adam MJ, Ammann W, Beattie BL, Calne DB, Martin WRW, Pate BD, Rogers JG, Ruth TJ, Sayre CI, Stoessl AJ: Positron emission tomography in patients with clinically diagnosed Alzheimer's disease. Can Med Assoc J 1986;134:597–607.
51 Haxby JV, Grady CL, Koss E, Horwitz B, Schapiro M, Friedland RP, Rapoport SI: Heterogenous anterior-posterior metabolic patterns in dementia of the Alzheimer type. Neurology 1988;38:1853–1863.
52 Jagust WJ, Seab JP, Huesman RH, Valk PE, Mathis CA, Reed BR, Coxson PG, Budinger TF: Diminished glucose transport in Alzheimer's disease. Dynamic PET studies. J Cereb Blood Flow Metab 1991;11:232–330.
53 Kuhl DE, Metter EJ, Riege WH, Phelps ME: Effects of human aging on patterns of local cerebral glucose utilization determined by the [^{18}F]fluorodeoxyglucose method. J Cereb Blood Flow Metab 1982;2:163–171.
54 Pawlik G, Heiss WD, Beil C, Wienhard K, Herholz K, Wagner R: PET demonstrates differential age dependence, asymmetry, and response to various stimuli of regional brain glucose metabolism in healthy volunteers. J Cereb Blood Flow Metab 1987;7(suppl 1):S376.
55 Mielke R, Herholz K, Grond M, Kessler J, Heiss W-D: Differences of regional cerebral glucose metabolism between presenile and senile dementia of Alzheimer type. Neurobiol Aging 1991;13:93–98.
56 Koss E, Friedland RP, Ober BA, Jagust WJ: Differences in lateral hemispheric asymmetries of glucose utilization between early- and late-onset Alzheimer-type dementia. Am J Psychiatry 1985;142:638–640.
57 Martin A, Brouwers P, Lalonde F, Cox C, Teleska P, Fedio P: Towards a behavioral topology of Alzheimer's patients. J Clin Exp Neuropsychol 1986;8:594–610.
58 Haxby JV, Duara R, Grady CL, Cutler NR, Rapoport SI: Relations between neuropsychological and cerebral metabolic asymmetries in early Alzheimer's disease. J Cereb Blood Flow Metab 1985;5:193–200.
59 Haxby JV, Grady CL, Duara R, Schlageter N, Berg G, Rapoport SI: Neocortical abnormalities precede nonmemory cognitive defects in early Alzheimer's type disease. Arch Neurol 1986;43:882–885.
60 Haxby JV, Grady CL, Koss E, Horwitz B, Heston L, Schapiro M, Friedland RP, Rapoport SI: Longitudinal study of cerebral metabolic asymmetries and associated neuropsychological patterns in early dementia of the Alzheimer type. Arch Neurol 1990;47:753–760.
61 Rapoport SI, Horwitz B, Haxby JV, Grady CL: Alzheimer's disease. Metabolic uncoupling of associative brain regions. Can J Neurol Sci 1986;13:540–545.
62 Horwitz B, Grady CL, Schlagter NL, Duara R, Rapoport SI: Intercorrelations of regional cerebral glucose metabolic rates in Alzheimer's disease. Brain Res 1987;407:294–306.

63 Akiyama H, Harrop R, McGeer PL, Peppard R, McGeer EG: Crossed cerebellar and uncrossed basal ganglia and thalamic diaschisis in Alzheimer's disease. Neurology 1989;39:541–548.
64 Foster NL, Chase TN, Fedio P, Patronas NJ, Brooks RA, di Chiro G: Alzheimer's disease. Focal cortical changes shown by positron emission tomography. Neurology 1983;33:961–965.
65 Haxby JV, Rapoport SI: Abnormalities of regional brain metabolism in Alzheimer's disease and their relation to functional impairment. Prog Neuropsychopharmacol Biol Psychiatry 1986;10:427–438.
66 Chase TN, Fedio P, Foster NL, Brooks R, di Chiro G, Mansi L: Wechsler Adult Intelligence scale performance. Cortical localization by fluorodeoxyglucose F18-positron emission tomography. Arch Neurol 1984;41:1244–1247.
67 Nestor PG, Parasuraman R, Haxby JV, Grady CL: Divided attention and metabolic brain dysfunction in mild dementia of the Alzheimer type. Neuropsychologia 1991;29:379–387.
68 Marsh JT, Schubarth G, Brown WS, Riege W, Strandburg R, Dorsey D, Maltese A, Kuhl D: PET and P300 relationships in early Alzheimer's disease. Neurobiol Aging 1990;11:471–476.
69 Polich JL, Howard L, Starr A: P300 latency correlates with digit span. Psychophysiology 1983;20:665–669.
70 Kumar A, Schapiro MB, Haxby JV, Grady CL, Friedland RP: Cerebral metabolic and cognitive studies in dementia with frontal lobe behavioral features. J Psychiatry Res 1990;24: 97–109.
71 Jagust WJ, Budinger TF, Reed BR: The diagnosis of dementia with single photon emission tomography. Arch Neurol 1987;44:258–262.
72 Johnson KA, Mueller ST, Walshe TM, English RJ, Holman LB: Cerebral perfusion imaging in Alzheimer's disease. Use of single photon emission computed tomography and iofetamine hydrochloride I 123. Arch Neurol 1987;44:165–168.
73 Ohnishi T, Hoshi H, Nagamachi S, Jinnouchi S, Fatami S, Watanabe K, Mitsuyama Y: Regional cerebral blood flow with ^{123}I-IMP in patients with degenerative dementia. AJRN 1991;12:513–520.
74 Hurwitz TA, Ammann W, Chu D, Clark C, Holden J, Browstone R: Single photon emission computed tomography using ^{99m}Tc-HM-PAO in the routine evaluation of Alzheimer's disease. Can J Neurol Sci 1991;18:59–62.
75 Johnson KA, Holman BL, Mueller SP, Rosen TJ, English R, Nagel SJ, Growdon JH: Single photon emission computed tomography in Alzheimer's disease. Abnormal iofetamine I 123 uptake reflects dementia severity. Arch Neurol 1988;45:392–396.
76 Jagust WJ, Reed BR, Seab JP, Budinger TF: Alzheimer's disease. Age at onset and single-photon emission computed tomographic patterns of regional cerebral blood flow. Arch Neurol 1990;47:628–633.
77 Burns A, Philpot MP, Costa DC, Ell PJ, Levy R: The investigation of Alzheimer's disease with single photon emission tomography J Neurol Neurosurg Psychiatry 1989;52:248–253.
78 Gustafson L, Brun A, Franck Holmquist A, Risberg J: Regional cerebral blood flow in degenerative dementia of non-Alzheimer type. J Cereb Blood Flow Metab 1985;5(suppl 1): S141–S142.
79 Gustafson L: Frontal lobe degeneration of non-Alzheimer type. II Clinical picture and differential diagnosis. Arch Gerontol Geriatr 1987;6: 209–223.
80 Neary D, Snowden JS, Bowen DM, Sims NR, Mann DMA, Benton JS, Norhten B, Yates PO, Davison AN: Neuropsychological syndromes in presenile dementia due to cerebral atrophy. J Neurol Neurosurg Psychiatry 1986;49:163–174.
81 Neary D, Snowden JS, Northen B, Goulding P: Dementia of the frontal lobe type. J Neurol Neurosurg Psychiatry 1988;51:353–361.
82 Mitsuyama Y, Takamiya S: Presenile dementia with motor neuron disease in Japan. A new entity? Arch Neurol 1979;36:592–593.
83 Morita K, Kaiya H, Ikeda T, Namba M: Presenile dementia combined with amyotrophy. A review of 34 Japanese cases. Arch Gerontol Geriatr 1987;6:263–277.
84 Brun A: Frontal lobe degeneration of non-Alzheimer type. I Neuropathology. Arch Gerontol Geriatr 1987;6:193–208.
85 American Psychiatric Association: Diagnostic and Statistical Manual of Mental Disorders, ed 3, revised. Washington, American Psychiatric Association, 1987.
86 McKhann G, Drachman D, Folstein M, Katzman R, Price D, Stadlan EM: Clinical diagnosis of Alzheimer's disease. Report of the NINCDS/ADRDA task force under the auspices of Department of Health and Human Services Task Force on Alzheimer's Disease. Neurology 1984;34:939–944.
87 Sam M, Gutmann L, Schochet SS, Doshi H: Pick's disease. A case clinically resembling amyotrophic lateral sclerosis. Neurology 1991; 41:1831–1833.
88 Risberg J: Frontal lobe degeneration of non-Alzheimer type. III Regional cerebral blood flow. Arch Gerontol Geriatr 1987;6:225–233.
89 Neary D, Snowden JS, Shields RA, Burjan AWI, Northen B, Macdermott N, Prescott MC, Testa HJ: Single photon emission tomography using ^{99m}Tc-HM-PAO in the investigation of dementia. J Neurol Neurosurg Psychiatry 1987;50:1101–1109.
90 Miller BL, Cummings JL, Villanueva-Miller J, Boone K, Mehringer CM, Lesser IM, Mena I: Frontal lobe degeneration. Clinical, neuropsychological and SPECT characteristics. Neurology 1991;41:1374–1382.
91 Folstein MF, Folstein SE, McHugh PR: 'Mini-Mental State', a practical method for grading the cognitive state of patients for the clinician. J Psychiatry Res 1975;12:185–198.
92 Jagust WJ, Reed BR, Seab JP, Kramer JH, Budinger TF: Clinical-physiologic correlates of Alzheimer's disease and frontal lobe dementia. Am J Physiol Imaging 1989;4:89–96.
93 Elfgren C, Gustafson L, Johanson A, Minthon L, Passant V, Risberg J: Cognitive function in dementia of Alzheimer type and frontal lobe dementia related to regional cerebral blood flow. J Cereb Blood Flow Metab 1991;11(suppl 2):S176.
94 Chase TN, Burrows GH, Mohr E: Cortical glucose utilization patterns in primary degenerative dementias of the anterior and posterior type. Arch Geront Geriatr 1987;6:289–297.
95 Kitamura S, Araki T, Sakamoto S, Iio M, Terashi A: Cerebral blood flow and cerebral oxygen metabolism in patients with dementia of frontal lobe type. Rinsho Shinkeigaku 1990;30: 1171–1175.
96 Belliveau JW, Kennedy DN, McKinstry RC, Buchbinder BR, Weisskopf RM, Cohen MS, Vevea JM, Brady TJ, Rosen BR: Functional mapping of the human visual cortex by magnetic resonance imaging. Science 1991;254: 716–719.
97 Majocha RE, Reno JM, Friedland RP, VanHaight C, Leon RL, Marotta CA: Development of a monoclonal antibody specific for β/A4 amyloid in Alzheimer's disease brain for application to in vivo imaging of amyloid angiopathy. J Nucl Med 1992;33:2184–2189.
98 Lezak MD: Neuropsychological Assessment, ed 2. New York, Oxford University Press, 1983.

Dementia 1993;4:204–213

Bruce L. Miller[a]
Linda Chang[a]
Ismael Mena[b]
Kyle Boone[c]
Ira M. Lesser[c]

Departments of
[a] Neurology,
[b] Radiology, Division of Nuclear Medicine, and
[c] Psychiatry, Harbor-UCLA Medical Center, Los Angeles, Calif., USA

Progressive Right Frontotemporal Degeneration: Clinical, Neuropsychological and SPECT Characteristics

Key Words
Right frontotemporal degeneration
Single photon emission computerized tomography

Abstract
The behavioral, neuropsychological and single photon emission computerized tomography characteristics of 5 patients with progressive degeneration of the right hemisphere are described. In all, the brain regions with greatest involvement were right-frontal and temporal. Psychosis, compulsions and behavioral disinhibition were the dominant, and often first, symptoms. Affect was flattened and the patients seemed distant and remote. Neuropsychological testing did not reveal a consistent pattern that helped localize the abnormality to the right frontotemporal region. These patients contrast dramatically to those with left frontotemporal degeneration in whom behavior and psychiatric status is often normal. This study suggests that the right hemisphere may be primary for the control of social conduct.

The First International Conference on Frontal Lobe Dementias of the Non-Alzheimer type was the earliest major meeting to explore the clinical, imaging and pathological features of patients with progressive frontal lobe degeneration of the non-Alzheimer type (FLD) [1]. Due to the imaginative longitudinal clinical, imaging and pathological studies from the research groups in Lund, Sweden, and Manchester, England [2–5], it is now recognized that patients with progressive frontal lobe degeneration can be diagnosed during life based on clinical progression and neuroimaging characteristics. More recently, studies from the United States have reported similar findings utilizing similar approaches [6–8]. These developments have led to improvements in the diagnosis of patients with FLD; patients in whom misdiagnosis was until recently extremely high. For example, a study of 21 patients in Minnesota with a postmortem diagnosis of Pick's disease revealed that 2 were diagnosed as Pick's, 1 FLD. Eighteen others were diagnosed as having Alzheimer disease (AD) [Mendez, personal communication].

However, the majority of patients with the clinical syndrome of FLD have pathological changes that are distinct from patients with AD. As was noted by Brun [1], the postmortem examination shows neuronal loss, gliosis and sometimes spongiosis. The characteristic findings of AD – neurofibrillary tangles and amyloid plaques – are absent. About 20% have Pick bodies and the question remains whether those subjects with Pick bodies have the same disease as those who show only gliosis and neuronal loss. More recent work by Snowden et al. [9] has found

Bruce L. Miller, MD
Department of Neurology F-9
Research Education Institute
1124 Carson Street
Torrance, CA 90502 (USA)

1013–7424/93/0044–0204
$2.75/0

that many of the patients with progressive focal degeneration of the left hemisphere have similar pathological changes to those with symmetrical FLD.

Numerous questions still remain about the etiology and pathogenesis of FLD. There are epidemiological clues including a dominant inheritance in some subjects and possible links with alcohol [8] and an association with amyotrophic lateral sclerosis [10, 11]. Although the clinical features of FLD have been described [2, 4, 5, 7], there is still a need for quantitative studies that correlate behavioral and neuropsychological findings with cerebral perfusion and metabolism as measured by SPECT and positron emission tomography (PET). For example, many patients with FLD develop semantic anomia. Yet, traditionally this aphasia is thought to occur when there is injury to the angular gyrus, an area that is largely spared in FLD [12]. Longitudinal, quantitative studies of cerebral blood flow (CBF) may help define correlations between behavioral and neuropsychological deficits and functional changes in specific brain regions.

The functions of the frontal and anterior temporal lobes in humans still remain mysterious [13], and FLD offers an in vivo model for the study of the clinical findings in patients in whom there is a progressive degeneration of anterior temporal and frontal lobes. One group of patients who may be particularly informative are those subjects with focal degeneration of the right or left frontal or temporal regions. A study of these subjects will allow comparison of right versus left frontal and temporal function.

There are extensive reports on patients with focal degeneration of the left frontotemporal region [9, 14–17]. Mesulam [14] first described this syndrome in 6 patients with a progressive aphasia without findings of a global dementia. The first manifestation of the language disturbance was anomic aphasia in 5 and pure word deafness in the 6th. 'Interpersonal conduct, social skills, judgement and insight remained intact, and some patients developed strategies for circumventing the language deficit.' In the few pathological reports available on patients with this syndrome the findings mimic those seen in patients with FLD; gliosis, neuronal loss and spongiosis [9]. Although there are many papers concerning left-frontal-temporal degeneration, there has been little written about the behavioral and neuropsychological features of right-frontal-temporal degeneration. We describe the clinical characteristics of five patients with progressive right-frontal-temporal dysfunction, all of whom differed dramatically on clinical and neuropsychological tests from patients previously studied with left-frontotemporal degeneration.

Methods

Clinical. The behavioral and neuropsychological characteristics of 5 patients (only 4 had neuropsychological testing) with dysfunction of the right hemisphere are described. Two were studied once while 3 others were followed over 2 years. In all 5 there was a clinical history of slowly progressive deterioration and SPECT demonstrated predominantly right frontotemporal hypoperfusion. The patients with right hemisphere dysfunction were chosen for description from a group of 30 patients with progressive frontal lobe dysfunction seen at the UCLA and Harbor-UCLA clinics. The majority showed symmetrical bifronto-temporal hypoperfusion.

All 5 were evaluated with the Brentwood-UCLA Neurobehavior Worksheet which assessed attention, language, visual spatial skills, memory, praxis and frontal-systems function. Laboratory and imaging studies were performed to rule out other causes for dementia such as hypothyroidism or stroke [18]. In patient 5, small white matter lesions on the right side and moderate-sized white matter lesions on the left were present. In none of the others was there evidence for cerebrovascular disease.

Neuropsychology tests included measures of gross cognitive function (Mini-Mental State Examination, MMSE) [19], intellectual level (WAIS-R Satz Mogel Format, verbal intelligence quotient, VIQ, performance IQ, PIQ) [20] verbal and visual memory (Wechsler Memory Scale-Revised) [21], Logical Memory (LM) and Visual Reproduction 30-min delayed recall (RO % Reten), Rey-Osterrieth Complex Figure (RO copy) with 3-min recall [22], language skills (Boston Naming Test, BNT) [23] and various 'frontal lobe' skills including the skill to shift and maintain set (Wisconsin Card Sorting Test, WIS CAT) [24], inhibition of habitual response (Stroop) [25], and word list generation (FAS) [26].

Magnetic Resonance Imaging. Brain MRI was performed in all subjects and the imaging findings were reviewed by a board-certified neurologist (B.L.M.).

Single Photon Emission Computerized Tomography. All subjects had a brain dedicated SPECT that allowed measurement of CBF with ^{133}Xe and high resolution imaging of CBF with ^{99m}Tc-hexamethyl-propyleneamine-oxime (HMPAO) [27]. ^{133}Xe provided an absolute measure of regional CBF. HMPAO gave high-resolution qualitative images of cerebral perfusion which were utilized for statistical analysis of regional changes in cerebral perfusion. A brain-dedicated unit (Headtome II, Shimadzu, Kyoto, Japan) with high sensitivity collimation was used. The system has 3 rings of 64 NaI detectors arrayed in a 42-cm diameter. Studies were performed with patients in the supine position, eyes opened and awake; ambient light and noise were kept to a minimum.

CBF was measured after inhalation of 30 mCi (1,100 MBq) of ^{133}Xe gas (Dupont, Billerica, Mass.). Sequential 1-min images each were gathered simultaneously for 3 slices during 6 min. Acquisition had 3 phases during which the patient breathed through a mouthpiece with the nose clipped: (1) Background acquisition performed for 1 min; (2) inhalation or equilibrium of 1 min duration of the ^{133}Xe and oxygen mixture; (3) washout phase of 4 min during which the patients breathed room air and exhaled into a charcoal-activated trap to retain exhaled xenon gas. Three transaxial images were obtained at 2, 6 and 10 cm above the orbitomeatal (OM) line after tomographic reconstructions with slice thickness of 2 cm. Images were extrapolated to a 128 × 128 matrix and displayed using a color scale coded to ml/100 g/min.

Table 1. Bedside mental status

Patient No.	MMSE	Word List	Drawing	Amnesia	Language
1	24	25 (FAS)	mild ↓	moderate	normal
2	30	2 'R'	normal	visual	normal
3	23	4 animals	normal	moderate	normal
4	22	2 animals	normal	mild	normal
5	21	9 animals	mild ↓	mild	normal

Table 2. Neuropsychology results

Test	Patient 1 1988	Patient 1 1989	Patient 2	Patient 3	Patient 5
VIQ	85	81	81	81	78
PIQ	70	66	85	–	72
Stroop, s	couldn't do	couldn't do	195	200	couldn't do
WIS CAT	couldn't do	couldn't do	0	–	0
FAS	25	21	4	0	8
Digit Span	8	6	4	9	8
Rey Copy	<10	<10	20	30	32
LM immed.	4	4	0	8	6
% Reten.	50	0	0	0	0
VR immed.	–	–	8	17	22
RO%, reten.	–	–	0	42	0
BNT	50	49	10	–	44
MMSE	24	18	30	22	21
Effort	fair	fair	fair	poor	poor

After ^{133}Xe studies, each patient underwent cerebral perfusion imaging with ^{99m}TcHMPAO (Ceretec™, Amersham, Arlington Heights, Ill.). They received 30 mCi (1,110 MBq) of ^{99m}Tc HMPAO intravenously via a butterfly needle. Scanning started 1 h after injection to clear soft tissue and muscle background activity. The same dedicated imaging device was used to gather simultaneously three brain slices 16 mm thick and separated by 32 mm. Acquisitions were completed in 30 min by shifts of 16 mm each that imaged the blind interslice space to yield 12 transaxial contiguous brain cuts. Transaxial scans were reconstructed in parallel starting at the OM line, and displayed with a color scale that defined the normal-to-abnormal interphase at 60% of maximal counts of all slices. 8 mm spatial resolution in the cortex and 9.6 mm in the basal ganglia were achieved. Coronal and sagittal slices were reconstructed to help study the temporal and frontal lobes. All ^{99m}Tc HMPAO images were evaluated qualitatively by the same neurologist (L.C.), blinded to hypotheses related to this study [28]. HMPAO quantification was performed on 6 consecutive slices; the first starting 1.6 cm above the OM line. A software package was used that automatically detects edges of the brain and divides cortex into 12 regions of interest (ROIs) in each slice. Mean pixel count per ROI was normalized to maximum counts of whole brain yielded a relative percent perfusion in each ROI.

All 5 subjects had quantitative analyses of cerebral perfusion performed in 6 of 9 slices from the transaxial images. Each slice had 12 ROIs. For statistical analyses slices were grouped into 3 slices and the ROIs were divided into 9 ROIs in each hemisphere. Accepting the potential limitations of statistical analysis with such a small number of subjects, we compared mean values from each ROI in the patient group with the same ROI in the 10 normal age-matched control subjects using Student's t test.

Results

Case Descriptions

Patient 1. A 56-year-old right-handed female developed progressive dementia associated with psychosis. Over several years she became more passive. Eight months prior to our assessment she developed the delusion that she had contracted AIDS through her husband. After treatment with neuroleptics the delusion diminished in severity but still remained. She became tearful and described depression. An obsession with her bowel movements developed and she spent hours in the bathroom. She spoke in obscenities and paced

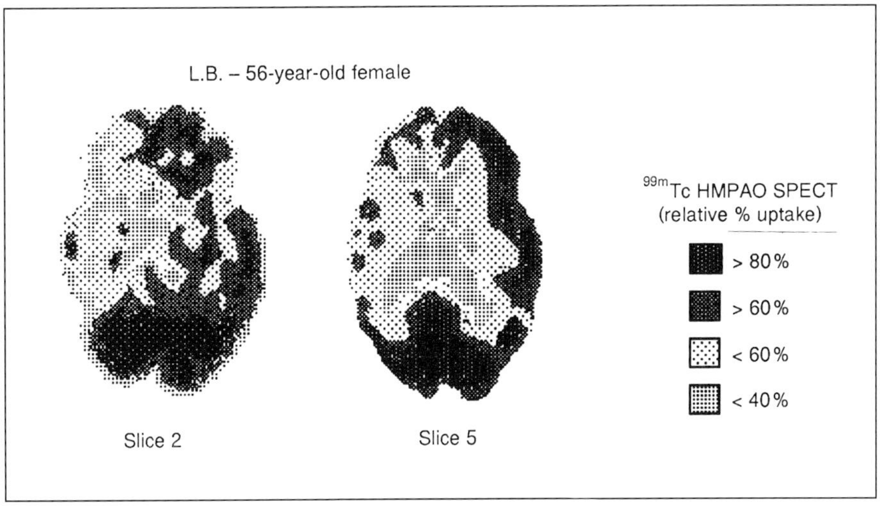

Fig. 1. Relative percent perfusion (as measured by % uptake of ^{99m}TcHMPAO) in patient 1. This figure illustrates severe hypoperfusion in the right frontal and temporal regions (both slices) and mild left frontotemporal hypoperfusion on the left (slice 2).

around her house. Often she attempted to hit her husband and he noted that she behaved like a 'robot' and seemed 'alien'. She changed from passive to aggressive during sex, started chain smoking cigarettes, gained 15 pounds and frequently spit. Memory worsened and she stopped reading or doing housework.

On examination she was irritable and anxious and often left her evaluation to smoke. She was diagnosed with major depression with psychotic features. MMSE was 24 and overall intellectual level was in the borderline range. Mild impairment was seen in attention, and selected language and frontal skills (word generation), with marked impairment in other frontal tasks, visual spatial skills, verbal and nonverbal memory. Basic neurological examination was normal. MRI showed mild right fronto-temporal-parietal atrophy. ^{133}Xe showed hypoperfusion in the right frontal (30 ml/100 g tissue/min; abbreviated 30 ml) and temporal (23 ml) areas with milder left temporal hypoperfusion (25–50 ml). HMPAO SPECT showed severe right frontal and temporal hypoperfusion with mild left temporal hypoperfusion (fig. 1).

She was treated with fluoxetine which alleviated the bowel obsessions and improved the irritability and anxiety. However, cognitive decline continued and memory worsened. One year later MMSE had dropped to 18 and every neuropsychological test showed a decline (see table 1 for mental status changes and table 2 for neuropsychology changes of all five patients.) The dementia progressed and nearly five years from the onset of her psychotic symptoms she was admitted to a nursing facility due to uncontrollably violent behavior at home.

Patient 2. A 60-year-old right-handed female was admitted to hospital after 1 year of progressive psychiatric decline associated with delusions. She complained that her problems started when a 'peculiar dentist' inserted radioactive material into her mouth causing her teeth to crack and abscess. She thought that she emanated radiation to others and called the fire department to clean the radiation out of her house's plumbing.

On examination she had a major depression with psychotic features. She was agitated and remote. Speech was circumstantial with loosening of associations. MMSE was 30. Comprehension was normal but there was a mild anomia. Neuropsychology tests showed a low average IQ. She named two 'R' words in 1 min and failed frontal tasks involving shifting set, categorization, and divided attention. Constructions showed omission of detail. Severe deficits were seen in attention, frontal skills and nonverbal memory. Basic neurological examination was normal. MRI showed generalized atrophy and few scattered white matter lesions. SPECT was not available at the time of the initial examination.

She left hospital with persistent psychotic symptoms. Over 1 year she became severely demented leading to placement in a nursing home. On examination at that time she was agitated and paced without interacting with the examiner. She was mute and MMSE was 0. ^{133}Xe showed CBF in the 35 ml range in the right temporal and parietal and left temporal areas. The left frontal region was in the 35–50 ml range. HMPAO showed severe right-frontal, temporal and parietal hypoperfusion. The left frontal and parietal areas showed milder hypoperfusion (fig. 2).

Patient 3. A 66-year-old right-handed female was seen for assessment of behavioral changes including loss of appetite, increased religiosity, irritability and social withdrawal. One year previously her eating habits changed and she became a 'picky' eater, losing 12 pounds. She began to express religious ideas that her husband considered eccentric. Her husband noticed increased irritability. She had increasing problems recognizing friends' faces and names but continued working. At work she became isolated and withdrawn.

On examination she was thin and placid. She had a flat affect and paced during the evaluation. She easily fatigued and repeatedly complained of feeling cold despite wearing several sweaters. MMSE was 23. Language comprehension was good but she could not name medium frequency words such as 'earring'. Even when told the word she did not recognize it. Word list was 4 animals. Calculation, drawing and basic neurology examination were normal. She had a borderline VIQ. Frontal systems, constructional skills and verbal learning were impaired, while non-verbal learning was average.

MRI showed a small lesion in the left parietal white matter. With ^{133}Xe CBF was 17–30 ml in the right frontal and temporal regions while CBF in the left temporal region was 25 ml. CBF in the left frontal area was 70 ml while the remaining brain ranged from 30 to 56 ml. HMPAO showed severe hypoperfusion of the right frontal and temporal lobes with moderate hypoperfusion in the left temporal lobe (fig. 3).

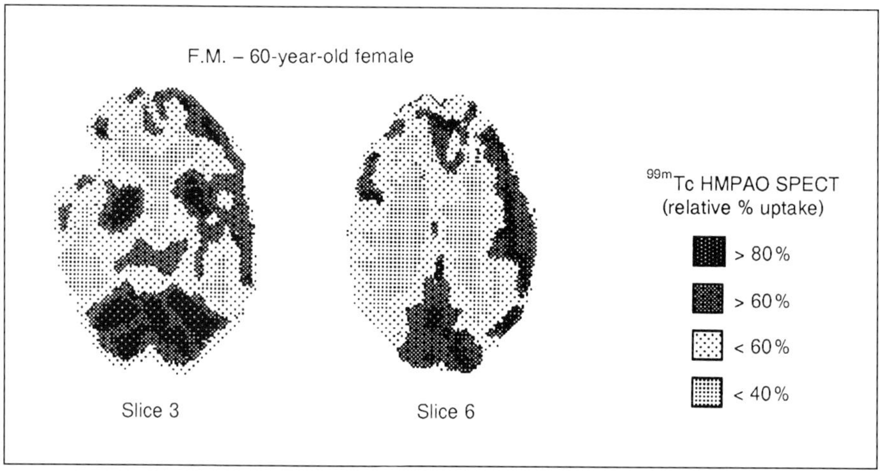

Fig. 2. Relative percent perfusion (as measured by % uptake of ^{99m}TcHMPAO) in patient 2. The slices illustrate extensive right frontal temporal and parietal hypoperfusion. Only focal frontal and parietal hypoperfusion occurred in the left hemisphere (slice).

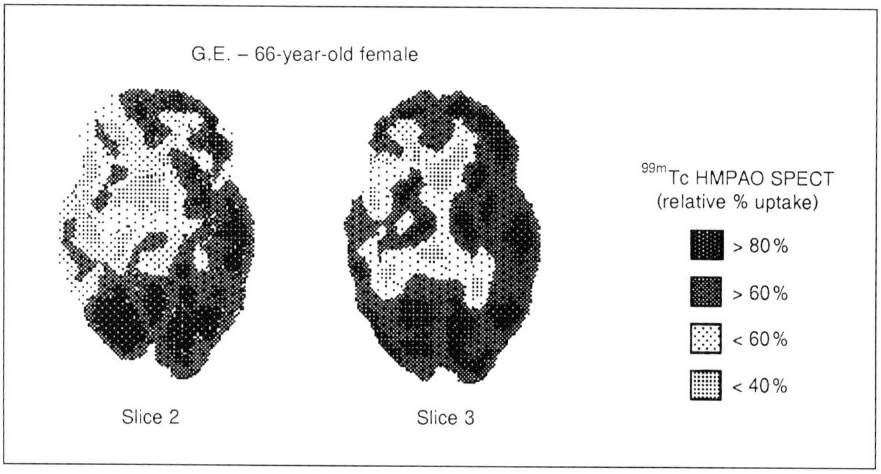

Fig. 3. Relative percent perfusion (as measured by % uptake of ^{99m}TcHMPAO) in patient 3. These slices show severe right frontal and temporal hypoperfusion.

Patient 4. A 56-year-old right-handed male began to inquire of family members how to get from one place to another. At work he made serious errors as an estimator, and without his wife's knowledge, paid back the company for his mistakes. He was gradually shifted to janitorial work which he could not do and he retired at age 58. Over the next year he exhibited 'silly' behaviors such as refusing to wear clothes, putting on different shoes and socks and placing deodorant and shaving lotion in his hair. He became argumentative with family and friends and developed a new interest in religion, spending much of his time in church. On examination he was placid and mildly irritable. MMSE was 22 with 5 points lost on orientation and recall and 2 lost due to the inability to name pencil or watch. Once he was told the name for the words he denied that this was correct. Digit span was 7 and language was normal except for a semantic anomia and an animal list of 2. He performed simple but not complex calculations and had normal praxis and hand sequences. Drawing was normal and neurological examination normal.

MRI was normal. SPECT showed blood flow of 22 ml in the right frontal and temporal lobes with mild left temporal hypoperfusion (30 ml). HMPAO showed severe bilateral basal frontal hypoperfusion with moderate dorsolateral right frontal hypoperfusion. Severe right temporal and mild left temporal hypoperfusion was seen (fig. 4). He continued to worsen and was placed in day-care where he was irritable and hard to manage.

Patient 5. A 68-year-old right-handed male became withdrawn and stopped socializing with friends. He lost interest in foreplay during sexual intercourse and his wife nicknamed him '1-2-3'. One year later he became passive and dependent on his wife. When he bought ice cream he would only order what his wife requested. He exhibited irrational behaviors such as taking apart a stamp collection and mailing the stamps on envelopes. He bought $17.00 worth of evening papers in order to obtain the coupons. He became obsessed with his urination, going to the toilet over 20 times every evening. He started urinating in public. While attending parties he would suddenly yell that he wanted to go home and he threw items out of his car window. Dietary habits changed and the only foods he desired were cokes and margaritas. He got lost in public.

On examination he was cooperative but indifferent and remote. Frequently he touched his groin. MMSE was 21. Speech and naming were normal. He generated 9 animals in 1 min. He remembered 0/8 words in 5 min after 3 trials but with clues got all 8. Calculation was excellent and hand sequences normal. Drawing showed mild impairment on three-dimensional figures. Neuropsychology testing showed IQ scores in the borderline range. Visual-spatial skills and attention

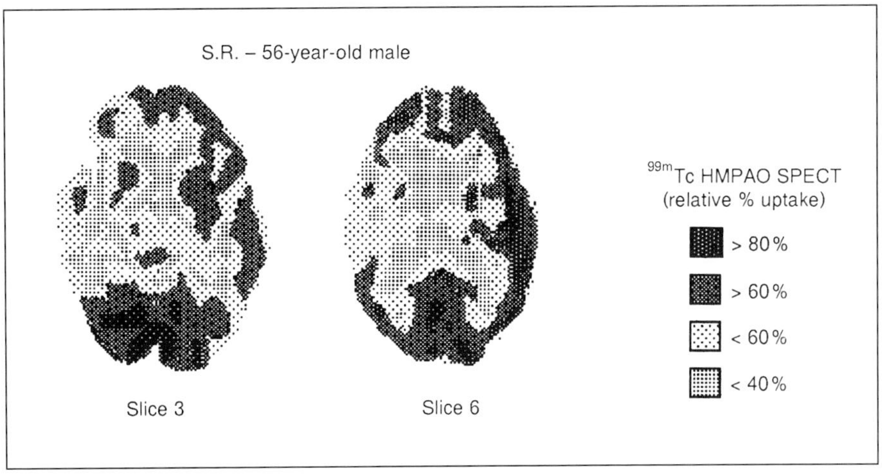

Fig. 4. Relative percent perfusion (as measured by % uptake of ^{99m}TcHMPAO) in patient 4. Severe right frontal and temporal hypoperfusion and focal left temporal hypoperfusion are seen.

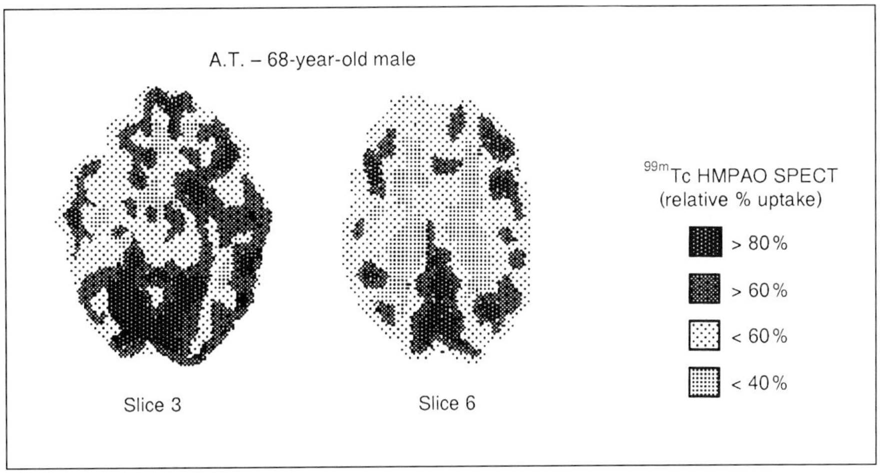

Fig. 5. Relative percent perfusion (as measured by % uptake of ^{99m}TcHMPAO) in patient 5. Severe diffuse hypoperfusion was seen through both hemispheres, right frontal and temporal regions are most affected.

were intact with mild declines in word retrieval. Marked deficits were seen in frontal and memory abilities. Basic neurological examination was normal. MRI showed small white matter lesions, primarily in the left-subfrontal and right occipital areas. ^{133}Xe showed severe diffuse hypoperfusion in the anterior portions of the brain with lowest levels of 30 ml in the right temporal and parietal regions. Occipital CBF was about 68 ml. HMPAO showed right frontotemporal anterior parietal and milder left frontoparietal hypoperfusion (fig. 5).

Summary of Bedside Mental Status and Neuropsychology Testing

The results of bedside mental status testing are shown in table 1. Of note the MMSE ranged from a low of 21 to a high of 30. Word list generation was severely impaired in 4 subjects and mildly impaired in 1. Drawing showed mild impairment in 2 subjects while it was normal in the other 3. All 5 had memory impairment which varied from mild nonverbal deficits to moderate verbal and nonverbal abnormalities. Language was normal except for naming which was impaired in all 5 subjects. In 4 subjects the naming deficit had the features of a semantic anomia.

Table 2 summarizes the neuropsychological findings. In general, IQ testing was in the low average to borderline range. Significant deficits were seen across both verbal and nonverbal memory. Impairment on frontal lobe tests was seen in all. In contrast, attentional skills and word retrieval were generally normal. Visual spatial skills were variable.

SPECT Findings. ^{99m}TcHMPAO: We found significantly decreased cerebral perfusion in the frontal and temporal regions in the right hemisphere but not the left (fig. 6). Of all the brain areas analyzed, the right anterior temporal regions had the most significant decrease in perfusion when compared to the normal elderly ($p = 0.0001$). In contrast, in the left hemisphere only one dorsal lateral

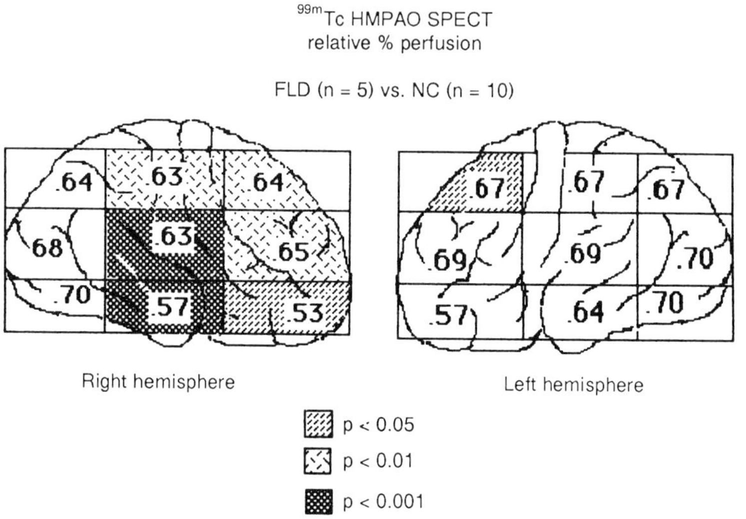

Fig. 6. Comparison of mean relative percent uptake in right and left hemispheres of FLD and normal subjects. There are many more significant regions of decreased cerebral perfusion in the right hemisphere compared to the left.

frontal region showed significantly lower cerebral perfusion in the left hemisphere of the patient group compared to the normal controls. When mean perfusion in each ROI in the right hemisphere was compared with the corresponding ROI in the left hemisphere within the patients, lowered cerebral perfusion was found only in the right temporal region (p = 0.008). We suspect that many nonsignificant statistical regional differences described here in the right versus the left hemisphere and the left hemisphere versus controls would have been significantly different if larger numbers of subjects were studied because differences in frontal and temporal perfusion were large with HMPAO (fig. 1–5) and ^{133}Xe measures also showed differences.

Discussion

Imaging and Clinical Features

We describe 5 patients with a clinical syndrome associated with progressive dysfunction of the anterior portions of the right hemisphere. In 4 of 5, the first evidence for clinical disease was a psychiatric syndrome, and all progressed to a dementia. In all 5 there was severe hypoperfusion of the right frontal and right anterior temporal lobes. Also, in every patient there was hypoperfusion of the left temporal lobe, always less severe than the right. In cases 2 and 5, mild left anterior hypoperfusion was seen. The clinical presentation in these patients was similar to that seen in patients with frontal lobe degeneration associated with bilateral frontal lobe dysfunction [2, 7], while the SPECT findings in the right hemisphere were similar (right frontotemporal versus left frontotemporal) to those seen in the left hemisphere of patients with progressive aphasia.

However, there were striking clinical differences between these right hemisphere patients versus those previously described with progressive aphasia. In most reports on progressive aphasia, the authors emphasize that social graces are spared and many patients continue to work despite having severe language deficits. In contrast to the typical presentation of progressive aphasia, all the patients with right hemisphere dysfunction had psychosis, disinhibition or bizarre behavior as an early or first symptom. At the time of presentation, patient 1 showed evidence for mild dementia while patient 2 had only a mild anomia. Eventually both were institutionalized with advanced dementia associated with severe behavioral disinhibition. A prominent component of 2 patients' symptoms (cases 1 and 5) was preoccupation with urinary or bowel movements. This unusual symptom was described by Snowden in 3 of her 14 patients with progressive aphasia [9].

Behavioral disinhibition or bizarre ideas and behaviors were early findings in all the patients. Irritability, verbal indiscretions, poor judgement and bizarre behaviors were common. In patient 5 sexual disinhibition was prominent, while patients 3, 4 and 5 had bizarre ideas and behaviors which included refusing to wear clothes, placing deodorant in the hair, newspaper hoarding, expression of bizarre religious beliefs, and throwing objects out of a car window. These types of behaviors are seen in FLD patients with bilateral frontal changes but are uncommon in patients with unilateral left hemisphere degeneration, even those with large areas of left hemisphere dysfunction and severe aphasia.

Another distinctive feature of these patients was the bizarre expression of affect. In 3 (1, 4 and 5) a major complaint of the spouse was that the patient seemed foreign or 'alien' and, in all 5, there was a remote, blunted affect. This abnormal expression of affect (aprosodia) [29] made social interaction uncomfortable for the examiners and for other individuals who socialized with the patients. The empathic feeling usually present in social interactions with early AD patients was absent in all 5, even those with normal or only mildly abnormal MMSE scores.

In patients 1, 3 and 5,elements of a Klüver-Bucy syndrome were present [30]. Patient 1 had altered sexual behaviors and hyperorality (weight gain, spitting and chain smoking), while patient 3 had changes in appetite and marked placidity which may have been early Klüver-Bucy symptoms. Patient 5 showed 'pet-like' placidity, altered sexual behavior and changes in eating. Why some, but not others, had Klüver-Bucy symptoms is unclear. All but patient 2 had mild hypoperfusion of the left temporal lobe yet patient 2 who had severe left temporal hypoperfusion had no Klüver-Bucy symptoms. Bitemporal hypoperfusion on SPECT was often associated with Klüver-Bucy symptoms, but bitemporal hypoperfusion did not consistently produce this syndrome. One possible explanation for the lack of correlation is that SPECT does not give sufficient resolution of amygdala and deep temporal structures to identify those most prone to develop the syndrome.

The most unique feature of these patients was the profound disruption of social conduct. This finding has potential implications for the understanding of hemispheric specialization. It is well known that the left hemisphere is responsible for language and reasoning skills while the right hemisphere is specialized for visuospatial processing. The findings in this small study suggest that the right hemisphere also may be dominant for the nuances of social conduct and interaction. Although disruption of social conduct is an invariable consequence of bilateral frontotemporal degeneration [7], typically it does not occur with unilateral left hemisphere degeneration. With unilateral left frontal dysfunction, behavioral changes do occur but these changes are often irritability, apathy or depression, findings that are distinct from those seen in our patients with right frontal dysfunction. In contrast, in the patients with predominant right-frontotemporal dysfunction psychosis, obsessive-compulsive behavior blunted or bizarre affect and behavioral disinhibition was present in all 5 patients. Although Tyrrell et al. [31] described a patient with focal right hemisphere hypometabolism in whom no psychiatric symptoms were present, the right frontal areas were largely spared. Blumer and Benson [32] and Eslinger and Damasio [33] have demonstrated that bilateral orbitofrontal injury leads to behavioral disinhibition. Perhaps, a major factor in the development of this syndrome of behavioral disinhibition is the right frontal dysfunction.

It is hard to attribute the behaviors described in these patients to injury in one specific area of the right hemisphere as all had hypoperfusion in both the frontal and anterior temporal lobes. In three patients right parietal involvement was seen (cases 1, 3 and 6) and in all there was at least mild left temporal hypoperfusion. However, the most prominent abnormalities in these patients were right frontal and temporal. It is possible that many of the symptoms may have been due to a combination of right-frontotemporal and left temporal dysfunction. The psychotic symptoms may have been generated in the right temporal or the combination of right and left temporal lobes [34] while the behavioral disinhibition may be attributable to right frontal injury [32].

Neuropsychological Findings

In these patients it was difficult to demonstrate that right hemispheric function was severely impaired based on traditional bedside mental status testing or with neuropsychological testing. One problem was that some of the patients were so uncooperative and behaviorally disinhibited that it was difficult to determine their true ability. However, despite this some patterns emerged. In 3 of the 5 drawing was normal, in 1 it was mildly abnormal and in another it was impaired. The sparing of drawing was probably secondary to sparing of the right parietal region and, in both the patients with drawing deficits, there was involvement of right parietal lobe with SPECT. All had decreased word list generation although the anomia present in all 5 undoubtedly contributed to this abnormality. Surprisingly, the Luria hand sequences [35] were normal although Benson suggests that the hand sequences are abnormal when there is frontal and caudate injury while with pure frontal disease they are normal [personal communication]. All subjects had problems with learning but nonverbal learning was often as compromised as was verbal learning.

Except for naming, language was normal. One surprising characteristic of the patients was the presence of a semantic anomia, an anomia that is thought to be associated with dominant angular gyrus injury [12]. However, the angular gyrus appeared normal with SPECT in every case. Due to the presence of semantic anomia and relatively normal right hemisphere functions, in cases 2, 3 and 4 it was predicted before SPECT that dysfunction would be more severe in the left hemisphere. Based on the findings in these patients it appears that bilateral anterior temporal injury can lead to this semantic anomia, even when the left-sided involvement is mild. This anomia appears to be extremely common in patients with many of the variants of FLD an observation made previously by Geschwind [Benson, personal communication].

The patients in this study performed poorly on memory and frontal systems tasks. Despite the fact that right-temporal involvement was more severe in all patients, both verbal and nonverbal memory were severely impaired in all subjects. This is probably explained by the fact that there are currently few good tests that help to distinguish right frontal from left frontal injury or right anterior right from left anterior temporal dysfunction [29]. The failure of traditional neuropsychological testing to differentiate right from left frontotemporal dysfunctions suggests that different neuropsychological tests, possibly those that quantify affect, need to be developed [29, 36].

The findings in this study suggest that right hemisphere degeneration should be considered as a diagnosis in patients with the late-life onset of psychotic depression, obsessions, bizarre behaviors, behavioral disinhibition or remote affect. Bizarre behaviors have recently been described in a small subset of patients with 'progressive language disorder due to lobar atrophy', although in some of those with this finding bilateral structural or functional changes were evident with CT or SPECT [11]. This suggests left hemisphere dysfunction may contribute to these behaviors.

This group of patients present an exciting set of clinical and neuropsychological changes. In all cases the symptoms were new in onset late in life and could probably be attributed to progressive brain disease. Statistical analyses of specific symptoms in larger numbers of patients with right, left and bilateral frontotemporal degeneration might help to determine the brain areas responsible for the behaviors seen in these patients. One potentially exciting approach to these symptom complexes might be to study the progression of symptoms and to correlate progression of brain disease with SPECT or PET.

Acknowledgements

The authors wish to thank Dr. D. Frank Benson who discussed many aspects of frontal lobe function and language with Dr. Miller. Dr. Jeffrey Cummings was valuable in helping formulate concepts related to organic psychosis.

This paper was supported by the UCLA Alzheimer Disease Center AG-10123-01, Harbor-UCLA's NIMH Center for the Psychobiology of Ethnicity and a grant from the NIMH, NH5567-02. Steve Read, MD, referred patient 4.

References

1 Brun A: Frontal lobe degeneration of non-Alzheimer type. I. Neuropathology. Arch Gerontol Geriatr 1987;6:193–208.
2 Gustafson L: Frontal lobe degeneration of non-Alzheimer type. II. Clinical picture and differential diagnosis. Arch Gerontol Geriatr 1987;6: 209–223.
3 Neary D, Snowden JS, Shields RA: Single photon emission tomography using ^{99m}Tc-HMPAO in the investigation of dementia. J Neurol Neurosurg Psychiatry 1987;50:1101–1109.
4 Neary D, Snowden JS, Northen B, Goulding P: Dementia of frontal lobe type. J Neurol Neurosurg Psychiatry 1988;51:353–361.
5 Cummings JL, Duchen LW: Kluver-Bucy syndrome in Pick disease: Clinical and pathologic correlations. Neurology 1981;31:1415–1422.
6 Knopman DS, Mastri AR, Frey WH, Sung JH, Ruston T: Dementia lacking distinctive histologic features: A common non-Alzheimer degenerative dementia. Neurology 1990;40:251–256.
7 Miller BL, Cummings JL, Villanueva-Meyer J, Boone K, Mehringer CM, Lesser IM, Mena I: Frontal lobe degeneration: Clinical, neuropsychological and SPECT characteristics. Neurology 1991;41:1374–1382.
8 Mendez MF, Selwood A, Frey WH: Neuropathologically confirmed Pick's versus Alzheimer's disease: A comparison of clinical characteristics. Neurology 1992;42(3):164.
9 Snowden JS, Neary D, Mann DMA, Goulding PJ, Testa HJ: Progressive language disorder due to lobar atrophy. Ann Neurol 1992;31: 174–183.
10 Salazar A, Masters C, Gajdusek DC, Gibbs CJ: Syndromes of amyotrophic lateral sclerosis and dementia: Relation to transmissible Creutzfeldt-Jakob disease. Ann Neurol 1983;14:17–26.
11 Sam M, Gutmann L, Schochet SS, Doshi H: Pick's disease: A case clinically resembling amyotrophic lateral sclerosis. Neurology 1991; 41:1831–1833.
12 Benson DF: Neurological correlates of anomia; in Whitaker H, Whitaker HA (ed): Studies in Neurolinguistics. New York, Academic Press, 1979, pp 300–314.
13 Stuss DT, Benson DF: The frontal lobes. New York, Raven Press, 1986.
14 Mesulam MM: Slowly progressive aphasia without generalized dementia. Ann Neurol 1982;11:592–598.

15 Chawluk JB, Mesulam MM, Hurtig H, Kushner M, Weintraub S, Saykin A, Rubin N, Alavi A, Reivich M: Slowly progressive aphasia without generalized dementia; studies with positron emission tomography. Ann Neurol 1986; 19:68–74.
16 Morris JC, Cole M, Banker BQ, Wright D: Hereditary dysphasic dementia and the Pick-Alzheimer spectrum. Ann Neurol 1984;16: 455–466.
17 Mendez MF, Zander BA: Dementia presenting with aphasia: clinical characteristics J Neurol Neurosurg Psychiatry 991;54:542–545.
18 Miller BL, Lesser IM, Boone K, Hill E, Mehringer CM, Wong K: Brain lesions and cognitive function in late-life psychosis. Brit J Psychiatry 1991;158:76–82.
19 Folstein MF, Folstein SE, McHugh PR: 'Mini-Mental State': A practical method for grading the cognitive state of patients for the clinician. J Psychiatry Res 1975;12:185–198.
20 Adams RL, Smigielski J, Jenkins RL: Development of a Satz-Mogel short form of the WAIS-R. J Consult Clin Psychol 1984;52:908.
21 Wechsler DA, Stone C: Wechsler Memory Scale. New York, Psychological Corporation, 1945.
22 Osterrieth PA: Le test de copie d'une figure complexe. Arch Psychol 1944;30:206–356.
23 Kaplan E, Goodglass H, Weintraub S: Boston Naming Test. Philadelphia, Lea & Febiger, 1983.
24 Berg EA: A simple objective test for measuring flexibility in thinking. J Gen Psychol 1948;39: 15–22.
25 Stroop J: Studies of interference in serial verbal reactions. J Exp Psychol 1935;18:643–661.
26 Benton AL, Hamsher K deS: Multilingual Aphasia Examination. Iowa City, University of Iowa, 1976.
27 Kanno I, Uemura K, Miura S, Miura Y: Headtome: A hybrid emission single-photon and positron emission tomograph for imaging of the brain. J Comput Assist Tomogr 1981;5:216–224.
28 Kanno I, Lassen NA: Two methods for calculating regional cerebral blood flow from emission computed tomography of inert gas concentrations. J Comput Assist Tomogr 1979;5: 216–224.
29 Ross ED: The aprosodias. Arch Neurol 1981; 38:561–569.
30 Lilly R, Cummings JL, Benson DF, Frankel M: Clinical occurrence of the Kluver-Bucy syndrome. Neurology;32(2):A9.
31 Tyrrell PJ, Warrington EK, Frackowiak RSJ, Rossor MN: Progressive degeneration of the right temporal lobe studied with positron emission tomography. J Neurol Neurosurg Psychiatry 1990;53:1046–1050.
32 Blumer D, Benson DF: Personality changes with frontal and temporal lobe lesions; in Benson DF, Blumer D (eds): Psychiatric aspects of neurological disease. New York, Grune & Stratton, 1975, pp 151–170.
33 Eslinger PJ, Damasio AR: Severe disturbance of higher cognition after bilateral frontal lobe ablation. Neurology 1985;35:1731–1741.
34 Cummings JL: Psychosis in neurologic disease: Neurobiology and pathogenesis. Neuropsychiatry, Neuropsychol, Behav Neurol 1992; 5(2):144–150.
35 Benson DF, Stuss DT: Motor abilities after frontal leukotomy. Neurology 1982;32:1353–1357.
36 Van Lancker D: Personal relevance and the human right hemisphere. Brain Cognition 1991;17(1):64–92.

Dementia 1993;4:214–219

C. Elfgren
U. Passant
J. Risberg

Departments of Psychogeriatrics and Psychiatry, Lund, Sweden

Neuropsychological Findings in Frontal Lobe Dementia

Key Words

Neuropsychological investigation
Primary degenerative frontal lobe dementia
Cognitive impairment
Cerebral blood flow

Abstract

Neuropsychological investigations were performed on 18 patients with a clinical diagnosis of frontal lobe dementia supported by regional cerebral blood flow measurements. Nature and degree of cognitive impairment were examined with a comprehensive test battery. The results of the neuropsychological assessment could be described as three levels of cognitive impairment. The increasing levels of cognitive impairment were accompanied by corresponding levels of reduced cerebral blood flow in frontotemporal areas. No apparent relationship emerged between impairment level and illness duration, indicating a considerable individual variation in the clinical course of frontal lobe dementia.

Introduction

The frontal lobes have rich connections, both afferent and efferent, with almost all other parts of the central nervous system. According to Luria [1] the frontal lobes, especially the prefrontal division, 'play a decisive role in the formation of intentions and programmes, and in the regulation and verification of the most complex forms of the human behaviour'. The role of the frontal lobes has been analyzed in numerous studies [1–6]. There is considerable agreement on the essential symptomatology of frontal dysfunctions. A mass of behavioral abnormalities have been described, including inattentiveness, inappropriate joking, tactlessness, distractability, or callous unconcern as described by Stuss and Benson [5]. Disinhibition, perseverations, and various forms of stereotypical behavior are frequently observed phenomena. The characteristic frontal lobe symptomatology is most clearly observed in frontal lobe dementia [6]. Examination of the gradual functional impairment accompanying the progress of dementia may provide insight into the structural correlates of frontal lobe function.

Degenerative dementia affecting primarily the frontal and frontotemporal cortex, without the histopathological features of Alzheimer's disease, has been described by Brun [7]. The frontal lobe degeneration of non-Alzheimer type is far more common than Pick's disease, accounting for about 10% of the neuropathological diagnoses in the longitudinal study of dementia in Lund [8]. Although the main distribution of the degeneration is quite similar in the two disorders, the morphological changes are different [9]. In dementia with early onset an even higher prevalence has been reported about 20% [10]. The typical clinical picture of frontal lobe dementia (FLD) has been described by Gustafson [11] and Neary et al. [12], and is characterized by a progressive personality change which includes behavioral disinhibition, stereotypy and socially inappropriate behavior. On clinical grounds it is not pos-

Christina Elfgren
Department of Psychogeriatrics
University of Lund
PO Box 638
S-220 09 Lund (Sweden)

1013–7424/93/0044–0214
$2.75/0

sible to distinguish between frontal lobe dementia of non-Alzheimer type and Pick's disease. We will use the abbreviation FLD for both forms of frontal lobe dementia.

Neuropsychological assessment of FLD has shown specific patterns. Johanson and Hagberg [13] studied 16 patients with postmortem verified FLD. Expressive dysphasia was the predominant and consistent language dysfunction, whereas reasoning and spatial functions were better preserved. Behavioral characteristics such as perseveration and confabulation were common.

The aim of the present study was to develop and to evaluate neuropsychological methods to assess the nature and the degree of cognitive impairment of patients with frontal lobe dementia, and in addition, to investigate whether different levels of functional impairment might correspond to different stages in the disease process.

Material and Methods

The selection of the patients for the current investigation was made in two stages. Out of a large group of patients referred to our psychogeriatric clinic, 30 patients with frontal lobe symptomatology were first selected. Then, on the basis of the clinical criteria by Gustafson and Brun [9] and Gustafson [11] used in previous investigations of FLD, patients with a presumed primary degenerative FLD were selected for further study. The validity of these clinical criteria has been established by the neuropathological findings of Brun [7] and Brun and Gustafson [8]. 18 patients thus conformed to the tentative FLD diagnosis. None of the patients had a history of cerebrovascular or systemic disease, drug abuse or indications of any reversible course of dementia. The diagnosis was further supported by regional cerebral blood flow measurements, using the ^{133}Xe inhalation technique and single photon emission computed tomography (SPECT) with ^{99m}TcHMPAO, SPECT showing flow reductions in frontal and anterior temporal regions. However, a definite diagnosis can only be obtained at autopsy. Four of the patients have died and 3 of them have undergone autopsy. The diagnosis in these three cases has been verified. The selected 18 patients varied in the severity of dementia. The mean age at onset was 54.7 years with a range of 39–70 years. The duration of illness varied between 1 and 13 years. Since the patients in the present investigation were expected to be at different levels of cognitive functioning we selected tests which were expected to be sensitive to a broad range of frontal lobe dysfunction. In addition, in order to see whether other more posterior regions of the brain were better preserved, tests which were assumed not to require complex frontal processing were also included in the assessment battery. The aim of the neuropsychological testing was to assess the following functional systems: motor functions of the hand, verbal functions, visuospatial constructional skill, memory functions, conceptual and executive functions. The source material for the tests and the description of the different tasks are presented in table 1. Regional cerebral blood flow (rCBF) measurements were performed using the ^{133}Xe inhalation method and a high resolution device [21]. The rCBF measurement was made close in time to the neuropsychological investigation.

Treatment of Data

Since no normative data for the Luria tests exists, the scoring is subjective and based on clinical experience. However, the tasks are, according to Luria and Christensen, within the grasp of any normal subject even at low levels of education. All test results have been graded on a 4-level scale (0–3) indicating the severity of the dysfunctions: 0 = no disturbance, 1 = slight, 2 = moderate and 3 = severe disturbances, or no fulfillment of the task. There are two tests in each task type (e.g. two tests measuring verbal memory and so on). The scores of the two tests in each task type have been summed up, resulting in a possible score of 0–6 in each task type. In order to be comparable with our treatment of the Luria tests, the results of the other tests were graded in the same way. This grading was made on the basis of the transformation of the standardized norms of each test, such that stanine 4–9 on the standardized tests were the equivalent of no disturbance which is zero on the graded scale (stanine 4–9 = 0, stanine 3 = 1, stanine 2 = 2 and stanine 1 = 3). In addition to the graded evaluation a qualitative analysis of the test performances was made, according to the suggestions of Luria. The statistical analysis of the neuropsychological findings was performed by Ward's method of cluster analysis, a multivariate statistical procedure designed to form groups or clusters of highly similar entities, minimizing the variance within each cluster [22].

Results

The variables that provided the basis of the cluster analysis were derived from each patient's scores on the sixteen cognitive functions. When determining the appropriate number of clusters we have used the procedure that examines the values of the fusion coefficients to discover a significant 'jump' in the values of the coefficients. A jump implies that two relatively dissimilar clusters have been merged, thus the number of clusters prior to the merge is the most probable solution [22]. This approach yielded three clusters. The number of patients in each of the three clusters was as follows: 5 patients in cluster 1, 7 in cluster 2 and 6 in cluster 3. The neuropsychological test results of the patients in cluster 1 are showed in table 2. Cluster 1 contained the patients with the mildest degree of cognitive impairment. Analyzing the motor functions of the hand there was none or almost no impairment concerning simple movements and complex forms of praxis. However in the tasks of dynamic organization the patients could not perform the taps or the reciprocal coordination of the two hands with sufficient smoothness, but they were able to correct their mistakes. Impressive speech in these patients was generally normal. Concerning expressive speech, however, there was a slight impairment in the nominative tasks, and particularly poor performance on the verbal fluency tasks, with subnormal frequency and some degree of perseveration. The patients had no difficulties with the copying tasks and the simple

Table 1. Description of the neuropsychological tasks

A Motor functions of the hand

1 Simple movements
  a Touch the fingers in turn with the thumb while counting them
  b Bring together, then separate the fingers of both hands, and repeat

2 Dynamic organization
  a Alternately clench and extend opposite hands
  b Tap twice with right hand, once with left hand and vv

3 Complex forms of praxis
  a Button and unbutton a shirt
  b Tie a knot and a bow

B Verbal functions

1 Word comprehension
  a Point to 5 named objects
  b Point to nose, eye, ear

2 Understanding of simple sentences
  a Point to the picture (among 5) which illustrates the sentence: 'The boy is reading a book'
  b Point to the picture which illustrates the sentence: 'The woman washes socks'

3 Nominative function of speech
  a Name 5 presented common, objects
  b Name from description eg: 'What do you call the thing with which you tidy your hair?' (3 different tasks)

4 Sentence construction, verbal fluency
  a Construct a complete sentence from three isolated words
  b Say aloud as many words as you can think of beginning with a specified target letter (FAS)

C Visuospatial constructional functions

1 Copying
  a Copy a square and a circle
  b Copy a 3-figure design

2 Visuospatial construction, simple tasks
  a Construct one 4-block design after demonstration
  b Construct 2 simple 4-block designs

3 Visuospatial construction, complex tasks
  a Construct 2 of the more complex block designs
  b Construct 2 of the most complex block designs

D Memory functions

1 Verbal memory
  a Retrieval of word pairs. The subject is presented with three lists of 10 word pairs each. Immediate recall is measured after each list
  b Recall of 2 sentences presented orally in succession

2 Spatial memory
  a The subject is shown 10 geometrical figures for 10 s each and is then asked to reproduce them from memory by drawing; number of correct scores are evaluated
  b The same as in task 2a but the number of error scores are evaluated

E Conceptual and executive functions

1 Thematic pictures and picture arrangements
  a Examine a relatively complex picture and describe the message or story it conveys
  b Arrange a series of pictures illustrating a certain event in correct order and state their unifying theme

2 Interpretation of proverbs
  a Explain the meaning of 2 proverbs
  b Choose the correct meaning of proverbs among several sentences

3 Different sorting tests
  a Object sorting test, 15 common objects are placed on a table in front of the subject; the subject is then told to sort the objects in 3 categories
  b Wisconsin Card Sorting test; administration according to Heaton

4 Maze tracing
  a The subject is told to trace a maze without lifting the pencil and without entering any blind alleys; four of the easiest items are given
  b The same as in E4a but four of the most difficult items are given

Luria's neuropsychological investigation [14]. Tasks: A1–B4a;D1b;E1–E2.
The Controlled Oral Word Association Test [15]. Task: B4b.
The Visual Retention Test [16]. Tasks: C1b;D2.
The Block Design Test [17]. Tasks: C2–C3.
Word Pairs [18]. Task: D1a.
Object Sorting Test [modified by Elfgren, 1991]. Task: E3a.
Wisconsin Card Sorting Test [19]. Task: E3b.
The Wechsler Intelligence Scale For Children, subtest. [20]. Tasks: E4.

Table 2. Median value and interquartile range (IQR) for the 16 cognitive functions in the three-cluster solution

	Cluster 1		Cluster 2		Cluster 3	
	median	IQR	median	IQR	median	IQR
Simple movements	0	1	3	4	6	0
Dynamic organization	2	2.5	6	0	6	0
Complex forms of praxis	0	0	0	2	6	0
Word comprehension	0	0	2	6	6	0
Understanding of simple sentences	0	1	2	4	6	0
The nominative function of speech	0	3.5	5	4	6	0
Verbal fluency, sent. construction	4	4	6	0	6	0
Copying	0	0	3	4	6	0
Visuospatial constr, simple tasks	0	1	6	1	6	0
Visuospatial constr, complex tasks	2	4.5	6	0	6	0
Retrieval of word pairs and sent.	4	2.5	6	0	6	0
Spatial memory	3	2.5	6	1	6	0
Them. pict. and pict. arrangements	4	5	6	0	6	0
Interpretation of proverbs	6	3	6	0	6	0
Different sorting tests	4	1.5	6	0	6	0
Maze tracing	2	1.5	6	0	6	0

IQR = Interquartile range.

visuospatial constructional tasks. However, there was a slight impairment on the more complex tasks. Organizational and planning deficits were observed. Concerning spatial memory, moderate impairment was observed and even more pronounced impairment was seen on verbal memory tasks. Confabulations were rather frequent. When dealing with conceptual and executive tasks the patients had obvious difficulties, none of these items were performed normally. Concerning thematic pictures and picture arrangements, the patients generally performed poorly. When asked to tell the meaning of a thematic picture they often gave answers based on their first visual fixation. When performing the picture arrangement tasks the patients first tended to leave many of the pictures in the presented order. However, when reminded of the rules, the patients did display some ability to correct their mistakes. The ability to understand the metaphorical meaning of proverbs was particularly disturbed. When the patients were instructed to select the meaning of a proverb they often regarded all sentences equally suitable for expressing the meaning. In the category of different sorting tests the performance on the object sorting test was normal while the performance on WCST was poor. Most of the patients could detect and verbalize different sorting principles, although they persisted in sorting according to a particular principle after it had ceased to be appropriate, in other words, perseveration. The performance on the maze test was slightly impaired. Summarizing the pattern of dysfunctions in cluster 1 the most distinct impairments were observed in the conceptual and executive functions. In addition there were some moderate impairments in the memory functions, the verbal fluency tasks, and in the tasks of dynamic organization.

In cluster 2 all the impairments of cluster 1 were present, but to a more pronounced degree (table 2). In addition, a slight dysfunction was observed in other areas such as impressive speech. Furthermore, coping ability was deteriorated and in addition severe impairment on the visuospatial constructional tasks was observed.

The qualitative evaluation showed additional types of errors. In the task of dynamic organization of the hand, the patients often tapped haphazardly and did not correct their mistakes. There was still no problem with the complex forms of praxis. Concerning the verbal tasks, there were much more perseverations and confabulations. The patients were severely deteriorated in the tasks assessing conceptual and executive functions, and had difficulty in both understanding and carrying out instructions.

The patients of cluster 3 were severely impaired on all tasks, and they scored 6 on each test (table 2). They were almost completely mute. Half of the patients in this cluster showed a utilization behavior, 'the tactile, and visual presentation of objects compelled the patients to grasp and use them', as described by Lhermitte [23]. In addi-

Table 3. Demographic data for frontal lobe dementia patients: A three-cluster solution

	n	Sex M/F	Age at onset		Illness duration (years) at exam		Level of education 7–9/10–12 years
			mean	range	mean	range	
Cluster 1	5	2/3	51.8	39–60	3.6	1–5	4/1
Cluster 2	7	3/4	59.7	41–70	4.6	3–9	6/1
Cluster 3	6	1/5	51.3	41–60	7.3	2–13	6/0

tion, they showed hyperorality. Table 3 shows the demographic data for the FLD patients in the 3-clusteral division. The sex distribution showed a greater number of females in each cluster. The age at onset was almost the same in the clusters. There was one patient in cluster 2 who had a very late onset, at the age of 70 years. Concerning illness duration, cluster 3 contained patients with an illness duration from 2 to 13 years. Some patients had almost immediately advanced to the most extreme level of impairment as opposed to others with a more gradual decline. We have also calculated the average rCBF pattern in the three cluster groupings, to see whether the different levels of cognitive impairment were parallelled by specific regional cerebral blood flow abnormalities. In cluster 1 there was only a slight flow reduction in frontotemporal regions, bilaterally. In cluster 2 the frontal flow reduction was more pronounced. In the third cluster, there was an even more pathologic flow distribution involving frontal and parietotemporal areas bilaterally.

Discussion

Our investigation of the 18 FLD patients, with this specific test battery, suggests three levels of cognitive impairment. The type of cognitive dysfunction shown here is similar to what has been commonly observed in patients with damages of the frontal lobes or thereby connected deeper structures [1, 3–5]. At the first two levels of cognitive impairment, clusters 1 and 2, the neuropsychological test profile clearly implicated disordered function of the anterior cortex, with relative sparing of functions of posterior cortices. At the third level, the patients were more severely deteriorated. The global impairment implicated not only frontal regions but also posterior areas. These group differences in distribution of functional disturbances were confirmed by the rCBF findings [24]. The earliest described manifestations of FLD are personality changes. All 18 patients showed personality changes in the preceding clinical examination. Blumer and Benson [25] have described two types of personality changes occurring after frontal lobe lesions, one toward apathy and indifference, and one towards puerility and euphoria, with mixtures of the two also being common. These two kinds of personality changes were observed in cluster 1 as well as in cluster 2. A comparison of cognitive performance between the three clusters would require that the groups are equivalent on all demographic dimensions. However, the distribution of males/females did not differ, and there were no notable differences concerning the level of education. There are some limitations to our study. For example, the interpretation of the data might have been improved by the inclusion of other dementia groups, like patients with Alzheimer's disease. Also, autopsy verified diagnosis was available for only 3 of the patients. However, that given these limitations we were able to discern three clearly different levels of impairment. In addition no apparent relationship emerged between impairment level and illness duration. This might partly be explained by uncertainty in determining illness onset but might also suggest considerable individual variation in the clinical course of FLD. One might even speculate whether the variations in illness course and impairment profile reflect etiological heterogeneity. However, there are other factors which may contribute to the individual illness pattern, like environmental and social conditions.

Acknowledgements

This study was supported by the Swedish Medical Research Council (grants No. 3950, 4969).

The authors thank Lars Gustafson, MD, Aki Johanson, PhD, Elisabeth Graae for constructive criticism of the manuscript, and Karin Nilsson, Anette Welin and Carina Wattmo for statistical and technical assistance.

References

1 Luria AR: The Working Brain – An Introduction to Neuropsychology. Harmondsworth, Penguin books, 1973.

2 Rylander G: Personality changes after operations on the frontal lobes. London, Oxford University Press, 1939.

3 Stuss DT, Benson FD: The Frontal Lobes. New York, Raven Press, 1986.

4 Fuster JM: The Prefrontal Cortex: Anatomy, Physiology, and Neuropsychology of the Frontal Lobe. New York, Raven Press, 1989.

5 Stuss DT, Benson DF: Neuropsychological studies of the frontal lobes. Psychol Bull 1984; 95(1):3–28.

6 Denny-Brown D: The frontal lobes and their functions; in Feiling A (ed): Modern Trends in Neurology. London, Butterworths, 1951, pp 59–84.

7 Brun A: Frontal lobe degeneration of non-Alzheimer type. I Neuropathology. Arch Gerontol Geriatr 1987;6:193–208.

8 Brun A, Gustafson L: Psychopathology and frontal lobe involvement in organic dementia; in Iqbal K, McLachlan, Winblad B, Wisniewski HM (eds): Alzheimer's Disease: Basic Mechanisms, Diagnosis and Therapeutic Strategies, Chichester, Wiley & Sons, 1991, pp 27–33.

9 Gustafson L, Brun A: The scandinavian view; in Hovaguimian T, Henderson S, Khachaturian Z, Orley J (eds): Classification and Diagnosis of Alzheimer Disease – An International Perspective. Göttingen, Hogrefe, 1989.

10 Knopman MD, Mastri AR, Frey WH, Sung JH, Rustan T: Dementia lacking distinctive histological features: A common non-Alzheimer degenerative dementia. Neurology 1990;40:251–256.

11 Gustafson L: Frontal lobe degeneration of non-Alzheimer. II Clinical picture and differential diagnosis. Arch Gerontol Geriatr 1987;6:209–223.

12 Neary D, Snowden JS, Northen B, Goulding P: Dementia of frontal lobe type. J Neurol, Neurosurg, Psychiatry 1988;51:353–361.

13 Johanson A, Hagberg B: Psychometric characteristics in patients with frontal lobe degeneration of non-Alzheimer type. Arch Gerontol Geriatr 1989;8:129–137.

14 Christensen A-L: Luria's Neuropsychological Investigation. Copenhagen, Munksgaard, 1974.

15 Benton AL, Hamsher K: Multilingual aphasia examination. Iowa City, University of Iowa, 1976.

16 Benton AL: Revised visual retention test: Clinical and experimental applications. New York, The Psychological Corporation, 1974.

17 Wechsler D: The measurement and appraisal of adult intelligence. Baltimore, Williams & Wilkins, 1958.

18 Cronholm B, Molander L: Memory disturbances after electroconvulsive therapy. Conditions six hours after electroshock treatment. Acta Psychiatr Neurol Scand 1954;32:280.

19 Heaton RK: Wisconsin card sorting test manual. Los Angeles, Western Psychological Services, 1981.

20 Wechsler D: WISC-R manual. Wechsler Intelligence Scale for Children – Revised. New York, Psychological Corporation, 1974.

21 Risberg J: Development of high-resolution two-dimensional measurement of regional cerebral blood flow; in Wade J, Knezevic S, Maximilian VA, Mubrin Z, Prohovnik I (eds): Impact of Functional Imaging in Neurology and Psychiatry. London, Libbey, 1987.

22 Aldenderfer MS, Blashfield RK: Cluster Analysis. London, Sage, 1987.

23 Lhermitte F: 'Utilization behaviour' and its relation to lesions of the frontal lobes. Brain 1983;106:237–255.

24 Risberg J: Frontal lobe degeneration of non-Alzheimer type. III Regional cerebral blood flow. Arch Gerontol Geriatr 1987;6:225–233(A).

25 Blumer D, Benson DF: Personality changes with frontal and temporal lobe lesions; in Benson DF, Blumer D (eds): Psychiatric aspects of neurologic disease. New York, Grune & Statton, 1975, pp 151–170.

Dementia 1993;4:220–225

Donald T. Stuss

Rotman Research Institute of Baycrest Centre for Geriatric Care;
Departments of Psychology and Medicine (Neurology), University of Toronto, Canada

Assessment of Neuropsychological Dysfunction in Frontal Lobe Degeneration

Key Words
Frontal lobe
Neuropsychology
Executive function

Abstract
The quality of the neuropsychological investigation of behavioural changes in frontal dementias is dependent on the specificity of the behavioural analyses. A review of methodological issues and published findings identifies possible potential reasons for misinterpretation of research neuropsychological data in these studies. The areas reviewed include the operational definitions of terms such as 'frontal lobes' and 'frontal functions'; identification of experimental limitations in frontal lobe research; and highlights of neuropsychological investigations of frontal lobe functions. These deliberations suggest a practical approach to the behavioural assessment of frontal dementias.

Neuropsychological Assessment of Frontal Lobe Dementias

In the past few years, degenerative conditions in addition to Pick's disease have been reported that have focal cortical pathology involving the frontal or frontal and temporal regions. As a group these disorders have been labelled frontal lobe degenerations or dementias [1]. These disorders have been defined by the type and locus of pathology in the brain, and as well by the behavioural correlates which have suggested frontal lobe dysfunction.

The differentiation of these disorders has been a significant advance in the scientific investigation of the dementias, and in acquiring the knowledge base to improve clinical care. To clarify further the behavioural specificity of these disorders, this review focuses on a conceptual approach to the evaluation of frontal functions and dysfunctions. The first section addresses the definition of frontal lobe functions and the underlying neuroanatomical correlates. This is followed by an outline of major methodological limitations in frontal lobe research. In the third section a selective review of recent experimental published reports allows the extraction of principles that should be considered in frontal lobe research. Finally, a practical approach for future neuropsychological research in the frontal dementias is presented.

Operational Definitions

Anatomical

The operational anatomical definitions of the frontal lobes and use of the term itself vary in different publications. For example, a classic text on the frontal lobes is titled *The Frontal Granular Cortex and Behavior* [2]. This title emphasizes the importance of the prefrontal cortex, as the frontal granular cortex is cytoarchitectonically defined as the area of the brain anterior to the premotor

D.T. Stuss, PhD
Vice-President, Research
Baycrest Centre for Geriatric Care
3560 Bathurst Street
Toronto, Ont. M6A 2E1 (Canada)

1013–7424/93/0044–0220
$2.75/0

region. Chapter titles in this book, however, also use generic labels, such as frontal cortex and frontal lesions. In contrast to the focus on the prefrontal region, the term frontal lobes in some publications may also denote a much greater area including all frontal regions back to and including the anterior cingulate. There is also considerable variability in the detail of anatomical analyses. Even though the frontal lobes comprise a significant proportion of total brain mass, estimated at 25–33%, published reports only sporadically differentiate the region of frontal lobes in question. Work by Barbas and Pandya [3, 4], Goldman-Rakic [5], their colleagues and others now identify significantly more specific architectonic differentiation and connectivity of the frontal regions. Yet, information on specific regions or pathways involved is only infrequently reported in human studies of frontal lobe-behaviour relations.

The frontal lobes, and the associated functions, also have been related to the anatomical concept of frontal systems and neural networks. The term frontal systems often indicates very direct and/or proximal anatomical/behavioural relationships, such as lie between the dorsal medial thalamic nucleus and the prefrontal cortex. There also have been suggestions of frontal systems that have less obvious anatomical connectivity. To date, these suggestions have derived from case studies of specific syndromes. Both Balint's and Anton's syndrome apparently present in a more fully developed and permanent manner if there is evidence of frontal lobe damage [6–8], suggesting that frontal dysfunction, either from focal damage to the frontal lobes or pathology in frontal-posterior connections, somehow contribute to these commonly regarded posterior brain syndromes. A more theoretical concept is that of neural networks related to a disorder. In neglect, for example, the frontal lobes are noted to play a qualitatively different role in the disorder that involves anatomically related regions.

Psychological

Does the term 'frontal functions' of necessity imply anatomical localization of function to the frontal lobes? Historically, the term 'frontal functions' evolved because specific disorders were best exemplified by lesions in the frontal lobes. In reality, 'frontal dysfunction' may occur for several reasons not related to focal anatomical disturbance. In a book dicussing the effects of ageing, Kinsbourne [9] writes 'A diffuse loss of neurons might handicap the victim in such general mental abilities as flexible problem-solving, the ability to change set and entertain improbable outcomes as possibilities, as well as to focus, maintain and then adaptively detach attention in a task', [p. 227]. The executive syndrome therefore may be considered a relatively common result of any global cerebral deterioration [10], even if transient and reversible. The symptomatology of acute confusional states, for example, has several parallels to focal frontal lobe disturbance [8, 11, 12]. Environmental factors may influence efficient performance in higher order tasks that have been considered 'frontal' tests. Sleep deprivation impairs effective performance on the Wisconsin Card Sorting Test (WCST), resulting in a lack of flexibility in the shifting of concepts [13]. Even normal subjects can exhibit dysfunction in executive 'frontal' abilities if demands of the task are properly manipulated [14].

Summary

Both the anatomical region of the frontal lobe involved and the psychological constructs of the function being studied need to be operationally defined when the frontal lobes are being studied. This is of particular importance in studying brain-behaviour relationships in frontal degenerative disorders. The concepts of localization, networks, and general brain dysfunction all may be relevant when trying to understand the behavioural disturbances which are considered 'frontal'. A parallel may be made with the behavioural changes that occur after traumatic brain injury. While the pathology in head injury frequently is predominant in frontal regions, the behavioural symptomatology with significant impairment in frontal functions may be related to multiple aetiologies, of which the focal frontal lobe disturbance is only one factor [15].

Some of the issues of defining the brain region involved in specific disorders and finding the appropriate behavioural reflection of this pathology are exemplified in a study that compared two groups of patients with dementia, both of whom met the standard clinical criteria for the diagnosis of probable or possible DAT but had different personality/social behavioural changes [16]. One group had significant frontal lobe features of behavioural disinhibition, and significantly decreased blood flow in prefrontal, orbitofrontal and anterior cingulate regions. The second severity-matched group of patients showed neither the personality changes nor the reduction in anterior glucose metabolism. Both groups, however, were similarly impaired on cognitive tests of frontal lobe functioning.

Scientists investigating the brain-behaviour relationships of the frontal lobes must consider that frontal lobe or executive functions as a psychological construct are not under the sole jurisdiction of the anatomical region called the frontal lobes: 'We do not mean to suggest that the executive functions, including cognitive programming, planning, and the maintenance of cognitive-behavioral selectivity, are not controlled by the prefrontal brain ... Instead, it is proposed that any diffuse brain dysfunction, affecting much of the brain to an equal extent from structural and/or chemical points of view, will disrupt executive functions before it will disrupt other functions' [10, p. 183].

Methodological Limitations

Several major methodological issues extracted from previously published frontal lobe research illustrate potential pitfalls in the study of brain-behaviour relations in subtypes of frontal dementias. The first issue is closely related to the specificity of the anatomical definition noted earlier. Patients with two general types of neuropathology have been used as sources of frontal behavioural symptomatology. One type produces relatively well localized frontal damage, such as that caused by vascular pathology and post-surgical states. The second type consists of those nervous system disorders which produce behavioural changes that are considered to be similar to those found after focal frontal lesions, as in multiple sclerosis and certain movement disorders. In this latter type, it may be questioned whether the observed behavioural alterations truly reflect focal frontal lobe dysfunction, frontal system disturbance, or cognitive changes independent of brain localization. The frontal dementias appear to fit within both categories, in that the pathology frequently involves the frontal lobes focally, but extends beyond.

There frequently is inadequate examination of the extent and location of the lesion in relation to the cognitive changes. Anatomically, the frontal regions have been divided into two or more anatomical regions, with suggested behavioural differences [4, 17]. The writings of Barbas and Pandya [3, 4] and Alexander et al. [18], and work by animal researchers such as Fuster [19], Petrides [20] and others have indicated that frontal abilities cannot be reduced to a unitary process. It is therefore important to isolate the anatomical region involved to help direct the selection of behavioural investigations and, conversely, to study which behaviours are correlated with particular brain regions.

Other methodological problems relate to small sample size because of the unavailability of patients with well documented disorders. The end result is inadequate sampling of data to ensure reliability of results both within and between subjects. The neuropsychological or cognitive evaluations may lack specificity. A review of the last decade of frontal lobe human research suggests that a significant advance in this time has been the attempt to isolate the specific component processes of frontal functions [21]. Many studies, however, continue to use clinical tests, or report experimental tasks which are often complex in order to tap cognitive resources that are not routine or overlearned, as patients with frontal lesions may show no deficits on simpler taks. These complex tasks often tap many abilities, hindering the efforts to differentiate and isolate cognitive processes.

Summary

Research in the functioning of the frontal lobes has been hampered by methodological limitations, many of which have been a reflection of the historical stage in the development of knowledge of this region, and a necessary consequence of the neurological conditions that affect this brain area. Awareness of these issues should lead to improved research in the neuropsychological investigation of the frontal dementias. The next section provides examples of why the development of the appropriate cognitive tasks is important.

Neuropsychological Investigation of Frontal Lobe Functioning

Several examples of published results in patients with focal frontal lesions are presented to illustrate principles of research in frontal lobe functioning that might be successfully adapted to neuropsychological studies in the frontal lobe dementias.

Studies in olfaction demonstrate the possibility of specific localization of function, and of proposing an understanding of how different brain regions may contribute to one disorder. Patients with intact olfactory bulbs and tracts but with lesions involving the frontal lobes have normal odour detection but significantly impaired odour discrimination [22, 23]. Patients with lesions in the temporal, frontal or dorsal medial thalamic region all were impaired in odour identification, suggesting a neural netword related to a function. Potter and Butters [23] interpreted the similar but milder deficit in one patient with a dorsal medial thalamic lesion as suggesting a hierarchically organized frontal system involved in odour-quality analysis. Among the patients with frontal lesions, only those with orbital frontal pathology had odour quality disturbances [22]. If monorhinal presentation was used, patients with left orbital frontal damage were impaired with ipsilateral (left nostril) presentation [24]. A lesion in the right orbital frontal area, on the other hand, resulted in a bilateral deficit. Proper patient documentation and directed test procedures led to data suggesting localization specificity both within the frontal lobes and between the two hemispheres, and a model of organization of olfactory functioning within the brain.

Attentional tasks provide another example of more precise differentiation of frontal lobe dysfunction. Salmaso and Denes [25], using signal detection analysis of a target identification task, found that patients with posterior lesions performed equivalently to control subjects. Patients with frontal lesions, however, were more willing to guess (liberal criterion level), and were less able to distinguish signals from non-signals. In another target detection task, patients with right dorsal lateral prefrontal lesions had particular deficit in the control of auditory sustained attention [26]. Wilkins et al. [27] also reported greatest impairment in patients with right frontal lesions in voluntarily sustaining attention. By contrasting fast and slow rates of presentation of stimuli, these authors were able to differentiate the basic ability in completing the task (no impairment at fast rate of presentation) from the sustained attention deficit (impairment at the slow rate of presentation). This selective review of attentional deficits in frontal lobe patients illustrates many principles: the possibility of localization of function within the frontal lobes; the importance of defining and using tasks that isolate specific cognitive processes, and the benefit of controlling for more general impairment that could confound interpretation of results of the frontal tests.

Studies on hypothesis formation, sorting, and shifting have provoked considerable debate about the role of the frontal lobes in such tasks. The WCST is commonly used, and is considered an important indicator of frontal lobe dysfunction. There now is question about the specificity and to some degree sensitivity of this test in identifying frontal lobe pathology. In many published studies, there was considerable overlap in performance between frontal and non-frontal patients, or those with diffuse pathology, even though group differences were significant [28–31]. A similar variability was noted in another hypothesis sampling test, the Levine Concept Formation Test [32]. Studies that did show a relationship between the WCST and frontal lobe damage apparently assessed patients in more acute stages of recovery. Certain case studies have reported patients with significant frontal lobe damage who performed normally on many cognitive frontal lobe tests such as the WCST [33–36]. In these case studies, however, the evident behavioural changes became obvious in social contexts or if on-line processing and time-limited planning and decision making were required.

Summary

Neuropsychological tests must be interpreted with caution in the study of behavioural changes after frontal lobe damage. Several reasons are likely responsible for the controversy in the literature. First, lesion locus may play a role suggesting a more specific brain-behaviour correlation within the frontal lobe [37]. Second, the cognitive processes underlying these tests are likely multi-faceted and these processes need to be dissociated. Subjects may fail complex tasks for many reasons and the relation of the test to a focal brain region becomes tenuous. Third, more complex tasks are likely to be disrupted by even non-neurological conditions, as noted above. Considering all of these factors, it therefore seems reasonable, and is suggested by the research findings, that a lesion anywhere in the brain might have some effects on many of the tests of executive abilities. Finally, sample size and data sampling are often too limited to provide adequate reliability and validity assessment.

These results do not deny the sensitivity and specificity of the 'frontal tests' in detecting frontal lobe damage. The data do indicate that these tests should not be used alone to identify the presence or absence of frontal lobe damage. Progress would also likely be accelerated if the cognitive processes selected were more specific; if tests were selected to tap the possible localization of abilities within the frontal lobes; and if the type of abilities assessed were broadened, including social/personality variables.

A Practical Approach

Many of these suggestions relate more pertinently to research with focal lesion patients, but are nevertheless relevant to the investigation of behavioural changes with frontal lobe dementia. Two general conclusions are proposed. The awareness that executive abilities are not under the sole jurisdiction of an anatomical region labelled the frontal lobes should create an appropriate scepticism in correlating brain and behaviour. This awareness also provides an opportunity for extending research in executive function by investigating whether there are similarities or differences created by different 'causes' of executive disorder. For example, is there an exact parallel with only quantitative differences in the effects of lesions in the frontal lobes or the dorsal medial thalamus, or are there qualitative differences? To achieve this, careful documentation of the aetiology of the disorder, the locus of the lesion, the extent of behavioural changes, and the environmental context is important. For the dementias, the stage of the disease may well be relevant, as is chronicity for acquired lesions. Selection of the tasks and behaviours to be assessed, and how they are to be analyzed, is important. Neary et al. [38] argued that patients with frontal dementias had a disproportionate amount of deficit in frontal lobe mediated neuropsychological functions than did patients with DAT. Kumar et al. [16], on the other hand, argued that personality changes were more sensitive indicators than standard neuropsychological tests of frontal lobe functioning, as these personality changes correlated with the decrease in blood flow in their study. In light of the recent neuropsychological literature it is recommended that both the specificity of the process and the severity of the dysfunction be carefully assessed, and these be correlated to the defined structural, metabolic, and/or biochemical alterations caused by the disorder. The goal of this review has been the clarification of the behavioural specificity of the frontal dementias. The development of systematic studies of the cognitive and behavioural changes is only now being initiated [39]. In addressing these complex issues, researchers and clinicians in the frontal dementias will not only advance the scientific understanding of the disorders and improve the care of patients with these dementias, but they will also advance the study of the functions of the frontal lobes.

Acknowledgements

This manuscript was prepared while the research of the author was funded by the Ontario Mental Health Foundation, and the Alzheimer Society of Canada. P. Mathews is thanked for typing the manuscript.

References

1 Cummings JL, Benson DF: Dementia: A Clinical Approach, ed 2. Boston, Butterworth-Heinemann, 1992.
2 Warren JM, Akert K (eds): The Frontal Granular Cortex and Behavior. New York, McGraw-Hill, 1964.
3 Barbas H, Pandya DN: Patterns of connections of the prefrontal cortex in the rhesus monkey associated with cortical architecture; in Levin HS, Eisenberg HM, Benton AL (eds): Frontal Lobe Function and Dysfunction. New York, Oxford University Press, 1991, pp 35–58.
4 Pandya DN, Barnes CL: Architecture and connections of the frontal lobe; in Perecman E (ed): The Frontal Lobes Revisited. New York, IRBN Press, 1987, pp 41–72.
5 Goldman-Rakic PS: Circuitry of primate prefrontal cortex and regulation of behavior by representational memory; in Plum F (ed): Handbook of Physiology: Nervous System. V: Higher Functions of the Brain. Bethesda, American Physiological Society, 1987, pp 373–417.
6 Hausser CA, Robert F, Giard N: Balint's syndrome. Can J Neurol Sci 1980;7:157–161.
7 McDaniel KM, McDaniel LD: Anton's syndrome in a patient with posttraumatic optic neuropathy and bifrontal contusions. Arch Neurol 1991;48:101–105.
8 Stuss DT, Benson DF: The Frontal Lobes. New York, Raven Press, 1986.
9 Kinsbourne M: Cognitive decline with advancing age: An interpretation; in Smith WL, Kinsbourne M (eds): Aging and Dementia. New York, Spectrum Publications, 1977, pp 217–235.
10 Goldberg E, Bilder RM Jr: The frontal lobes and hierarchical organization of cognitive control; in Perecman E (ed): The Frontal Lobes Revisited. New York, IRBN Press, 1987, pp 159–187.
11 Geschwind N: Disorders of attention: A frontier in neuropsychology. Phil Trans R Soc Lond 1982;B298:173–185.
12 Lipowski ZL: Delirium: Acute Confusional States. New York, Oxford University Press, 1990.
13 Herscovitch J, Stuss DT, Broughton R: Changes in cognitive processing following short-term cumulative partial sleep deprivation and recovery oversleeping. Can J Neurol 1980;2:301–319.
14 Moscovitch M: A neuropsychological model of memory and consciousness; in Squires L, Butters N (eds): The Neuropsychology of Memory, ed 2. New York, Guilford, 1992, pp 5–22.
15 Stuss DT, Gow CA: 'Frontal dysfunction' after traumatic brain injury. Neuropsychiatr Neuropsychol Behav Neurol 1992;5:272–282.
16 Kumar A, Schapiro MB, Haxby JV, Grady CL, Friedland RP: Cerebral metabolic and cognitive studies in dementia with frontal lobe behavioural features. J Psychiatry Res 1990;24:97–109.
17 Rosenkilde CE: Functional heterogeneity of the prefrontal cortex in the monkey: A review. Behav Neural Biol 1979;25:301–345.
18 Alexander GE, DeLong MR, Strick PL: Parallel organization of functionally segregated circuits linking basal ganglia and cortex. Annu Rev Neurosci 1986;9:357–381.
19 Fuster JM: The Prefrontal Cortex. Anatomy, Physiology and Neuropsychology of the Frontal Lobe, ed 2. New York, Raven Press, 1989.
20 Petrides M: Conditional learning and the primate frontal cortex; in Perecman E (ed): The Frontal Lobes Revisited. New York, IRBN Press, 1987, pp 91–108.
21 Stuss DT, Eskes GA, Foster JK: Experimental neuropsychological studies of frontal lobe functions; in Boller F, Grafman J (eds): Handbook of Neuropsychology. Amsterdam, Elsevier, vol 9, in press.
22 Jones-Gotman M, Zatorre RJ: Olfactory identification deficits in patients with focal cerebral excision. Neuropsychology 1988;26:387–400.
23 Potter H, Butters N: An assessment of olfactory deficits in patients with damage to prefrontal cortex. Neuropsychology 1980;18:621–628.
24 Zatorre RJ, Jonas-Gotman M: Human olfactory discrimination after unilateral frontal or temporal lobectomy. Brain 1991;114:71–84.
25 Salmaso D, Denes G: Role of the frontal lobes on an attention task: A signal detection analysis. Percept Mot Skills 1982;54:1147–1150.

26 Woods DL, Knight RT: Electrophysiologic evidence of increased distractibility after dorsolateral prefrontal lesions. Neurology 1986;36: 212–216.
27 Wilkins AJ, Shallice T, McCarthy R: Frontal lesions and sustained attention. Neuropsychology 1987;25:359–365.
28 Anderson SW, Damasio H, Jones RD, Tranel D: Wisconsin Card Sorting Test performance as a measure of frontal lobe damage. J Clin Exp Neuropsychol 1991;13:909–922.
29 Grafman J, Jonas B, Salazar A: Wisconsin Card Sorting Test performance based on location and size of neuroanatomical lesion in Vietnam veterans with penetrating head injury. Percept Mot Skills 1990;71:1120–1122.
30 Nelson HE: A modified card sorting test sensitive to frontal lobe defects. Cortex 1976;12: 313–324.
31 Robinson AL, Heaton RK, Lehman RAW, Stilson DW: The utility of the Wisconsin Card Sorting Test in detecting and localizing frontal lobe lesions. J Consult Clin Psychol 1980;48: 605–614.
32 Cicerone KD, Lazar RM: Effects of frontal lobe lesions on hypothesis sampling during concept formation. Neuropsychology 1983;21:513–524.
33 Eslinger PJ, Damasio AR: Severe disturbance of higher cognition after bilateral frontal lobe ablation: Patient EVR. Neurology 1985;35: 1731–1741.
34 Heck ET, Bryer JB: Superior sorting and categorizing ability in a case of bilateral frontal atrophy: An exception to the rule. J Clin Exp Neuropsychol 1986;8:313–316.
35 Shallice T, Burgess PW: Deficits in strategy application following frontal lobe damage in man. Brain 1991;114:727–741.
36 Stuss DT: Self, awareness and the frontal lobes: A neuropsychological perspective; in Strauss J, Goethals GR (eds): The Self: Interdisciplinary Approaches. New York, Springer, 1991, pp 255–278.
37 Milner B: Some effects of frontal lobectomy in man; in Warren JM, Akert K (eds): The Frontal Granular Cortex and Behavior. New York, McGraw-Hill, pp 313–334.
38 Neary D, Snowden JS, Northen B, Goulding P: Dementia of frontal lobe type. J Neurol Neurosurg Psychiatry 1988;51:353–361.
39 Moss MB, Albert MS, Kemper TL: Neuropsychology of frontal lobe dementia; in White RF: Clinical Syndromes in Adult Neuropsychology: The Practitioner's Handbook. Amsterdam, Elsevier, 1992, pp 287–303.

Dementia 1993;4:226–231

J.S. Snowden
D. Neary

Department of Neurology, Manchester Royal Infirmary, Manchester, UK

Progressive Language Dysfunction and Lobar Atrophy

Key Words
Progressive aphasia
Dementia of frontal lobe type
Lobar atrophy
Semantics
Phonology
Echolalia
Perseveration
Mutism

Abstract
The patterns of language disorder associated with 'progressive aphasia' due to lobar atrophy were compared with the language dysfunction of patients with dementia of frontal lobe type (DFT). The progressive aphasias were characterised primarily by impairment at the structural levels of language: phonology, grammar and semantics, whereas DFT was associated primarily with aspontaneity and loss of generative capability. However, there was overlap in language symptomatology, particularly with progression of disease. The findings lend support to the argument that progressive aphasia and DFT represent different clinical manifestations of a common pathology, and form part of the spectrum of lobar atrophies.

Introduction

Circumscribed cerebral atrophy may be associated with a progressive and relatively selective breakdown in language. Case studies have proliferated [1–14] and the clinical designation 'slowly progressive aphasia' has become widely used. It is recognized too that in the form of dementia designated frontal lobe degeneration [15] or dementia of frontal lobe type (DFT) [16], in addition to the characteristic alteration in personality and behaviour, changes in language function are a prominent feature. It has been argued that DFT, with and without the accompaniment of motor neurone disease, and progressive aphasia are different clinical manifestations of a common underlying pathology [14, 17 and see Neary et al., this volume], the particular characteristics of a given patient being determined by the topographical distribution of pathology. If that is the case, and progressive aphasia and DFT are not distinct entities, then one might predict some overlap in symptomatology both across patient groups and within individual patients with disease progression. Some evidence for this has been recorded with respect to behavioural changes: in progressive aphasia behavioural disorder and personality change may emerge with disease progression reminiscent of that seen in frontal lobe dementia [14]. In 2 brothers with an almost identical language disorder, early 'frontal lobe' behavioural changes occurred in one but not the other, differences mirrored by differential prominence of frontal lobe pathology in the 2 cases [Neary et al., this issue, pp 150–156]. Nevertheless, despite these suggestions of a clinical overlap, direct comparisons of the language disorder associated with progressive aphasia and dementia of frontal lobe type have not been drawn. The purpose of this paper

J.S. Snowden
Department of Neurology
Manchester Royal Infirmary
Manchester M13 9WL (UK)

1013–7424/93/0044–0226
$2.75/0

Table 1. Patient details

	Sex		Mean age onset years	Range	Duration illness years	Range
	M	F				
Progressive aphasia	12	7	61	52–71	9[1]	5–13
DFT	7	7	54	45–64	8	1–23
DFT + MND	5	0	55	43–67	2	2–3

[1] Based on 5 cases only.

is to compare the nature of language disorder associated with progressive aphasia and DFT. The presence of common features would provide clinical support for the view that DFT and progressive aphasia are manifestations of a common underlying disease process.

Methods

We have had the opportunity to study longitudinally 19 patients with a progressive aphasic disorder associated with a focal cerebral atrophy. Clinical details of 16 have been described previously [14]. All demonstrated an insidious deterioration of language, despite being physically well and showing no evidence of impaired visuospatial or day to day memory function. They have shown a circumscribed abnormality on SPET imaging, the distribution varying dependent upon the pattern of language disorder. Five patients have come to autopsy and the presence of circumscribed cerebral atrophy and non-Alzheimer pathology has been confirmed. We have studied approximately 100 patients with a clinical diagnosis of DFT, who presented with a behavioural and personality change similar to that described previously [16]. In all, neuropsychological investigations have highlighted frontal lobe dysfunction and this has been mirrored by bilateral frontal lobe abnormalities on SPET imaging. For comparative purposes we have selected those 19 patients for whom autopsy pathological data are now available, thus allowing confirmation of the diagnosis and also permitting evaluation of language to be based on the entire course of disease. In 5 cases the syndrome of DFT was combined with clinical findings of motor neurone disease [18]. The language symptoms in patients with and without motor neurone disease were similar so that they are considered together. The 19 patients would seem from our experience to be representative of the larger clinical group of DFT patients in terms of the features of language impairment.

Details of patients are shown in table 1. In both progressive aphasia and DFT there was a preponderance of males. Onset of illness was generally in the presenium, although slightly later in patients with progressive aphasia. Duration of illness was comparable, with a wide variation between patients, with the exception that patients with DFT combined with motor neurone disease had a uniformly brief illness.

Results

Profiles of Language Disorder

Progressive Aphasia

We have distinguished three broad patterns of language disorder: non-fluent, fluent and mixed.

Nonfluent. In the non-fluent group (6 patients) the predominant abnormality was in speech production. Speech was agrammatic, there were frequent phonemic errors, and sometimes a stuttering quality. The ability to repeat was severely impaired and the patient had difficulty naming and made paraphasic errors. Paralexic errors occurred in reading, and writing had a telegrammatic quality, with omission of functional words. Comprehension initially was only mildly impaired and the language difficulty was one principally in the domain of language production. The language disorder bore similarities to a Broca type of aphasia. With progression, output diminished and comprehension deteriorated. SPET imaging revealed reduced uptake of tracer extensively throughout the left hemisphere.

Fluent. In the fluent group (7 patients) there was a profound loss of word meaning, so that the patient could no longer name nor understand the meaning of words. In spontaneous speech utterances were produced effortlessly, but conveyed little information. There was a notable lack of precise substantive terms and patients tended to rely on broad generic terms such as 'thing' or else used certain words overinclusively. For example, one patient used the word 'water' to refer to all types of liquid, another used the word 'twisting' to refer to all types of movement including walking, and 'banging' to refer to all noises including the barking of a dog, reflecting loss of semantic differentiation. Phonological and syntactic aspects of language were well preserved, the patient could repeat and produce verbal or numerical series and carry out nursery rhyme completion, albeit without comprehension. The language disorder has characteristics of a transcortical sensory aphasia.

The abnormality lies predominantly at the level of semantics. In some of these patients semantic loss may be highly specific and appear to be more marked for certain classes of information. Of the 7 patients, 1 had particular difficulty in understanding animal terms, a finding described by other authors [19–23]. This finding is difficult to interpret simply in terms of the level of difficulty of test materials because it was not a universal finding among the patient group. Another patient retained the names of countries at a time when naming for other items was virtually impossible, a finding also described previously [24]. For example, when shown an outline map of Europe he correctly named Czechoslovakia and Bulgaria. In a verbal fluency test, when asked to produce words beginning with 'A' he produced only 'Austria, Australia and Azerbaijan'. When shown pictures of animals or buildings he consistently named the country of origin e.g. 'Africa', but was unable to name the test item e.g. 'lion'. The patient is now mute, so the effect no longer persists. These disparities are both intriguing clinically and important theoretically in terms of their implications for the nature of psychological mechanisms underlying meaning representation.

In this group of patients the semantic disorder gradually encompasses the visual domain, so that the patient no longer understands the significance of objects [25]. Five of the 7 have developed an associative agnosia. In keeping with this, functional imaging using SPET indicates reduction in uptake bilaterally in the anterior cerebral hemispheres, whereas in patients with a restricted verbal semantic deficit the left temporal region is affected asymmetrically.

Mixed. The first two groups may be regarded as two extremes: the one prototypical of a phonological disorder, with relatively preserved semantics, at least in the early phase of disease; the second a disorder of semantics with relatively preserved phonology. Six patients shared features of the two. Four patients had a non-fluent agrammatic speech, with phonemic errors, but this was combined with a profound disorder of comprehension. Two patients had a fluent output, and press of speech with comprehension disorder, with both phonemic and semantic paraphasias, reminiscent of a Wernicke type aphasia. Although naming disorder is generally regarded as pathognomonic of patients with progressive aphasia, its severity is variable. The 2 patients with fluent output were surprisingly good at picture naming.

Dementia of Frontal Lobe Type

The pervading characteristic was a gradual reduction in speech output leading ultimately to total mutism. Patients did not generate information spontaneously, and in response to questions responses were economical and often monosyllabic. There was little effort to produce an accurate response and responses such as 'don't know' or 'no idea' were common, particularly to non-automatic tasks requiring mental thought. The response 'don't know' was on occasions immediately followed by the correct response, providing evidence that responses may not accurately reflect the vocabulary potentially available to the patient. All but 1 patient had become totally mute by the final year of life. Verbal stereotypies occurred in 47% of patients. In general, these constituted favourite words or phrases. However in 1 patient, questions invariably elicited an irrelevant monologue of several minutes duration, in which minutiae of his daily activities were detailed. With disease progression, this stereotypy was maintained, although with gradual contraction of his restricted repertoire, and increased press of delivery. Aside from this 'record', he remained silent and did not initiate conversation. He alone had not become mute by the time of his death. Echolalia occurred in 47% of patients and perseveration of verbal responses in 100% of patients. In some, these features were marked and in one patient perseveration of writing was a presenting characteristic. Comprehension of language was compromised by (a) inattention and distractibility, (b) failure to adopt or shift mental set, and (c) concreteness of thought. General questions were frequently answered rigidly in terms of the subject's personal experience (e.g. Qu. 'Can you think of some names of animals?' Ans. 'Toby, the cat'. Qu. 'What other animals are there?' Ans. 'We've only got a cat'). Comprehension became more difficult to evaluate as the patient became increasingly unresponsive. The language characteristics of these patients are similar to those described by other authors [15]. The major characteristics of the language disorder in the non-fluent and fluent forms of progressive aphasia and in DFT are summarised in table 2.

Similarities between Language Disorder in DFT and Progressive Aphasia

Structural Aspects of Language in DFT

Aspontaneity and reduction in output leading to mutism were the overriding feature in DFT patients. The question arises as to the extent to which breakdown in

Table 2. Principle language characteristics in progressive aphasia and DFT

	Progressive aphasia		DFT
	non-fluent	fluent	
Spontaneous speech	Agrammatic		Reduced output
	Phonemic errors	Semantic errors	Echolalia, stereotypy, perseveration
Series speech	Impaired	Preserved	Reduced output
Comprehension	Mild impairment initially	Profound impairment	Concrete
	Worse for syntax	Loss of individual word meaning	Failure of mental set
Repetition	Impaired	Preserved	Preserved (cursory)
Naming	Moderate impairment	Profound impairment	Impaired
	Phonemic and verbal errors	Semantic errors	Omission errors
Reading	Non-fluent, paralexic errors	Fluent, some sound regularisations	Reduced output
Writing	Telegrammatic, spelling errors	Orthographic regularisations	Perseveration

structural aspects of language was also present, similar to that seen in progressive aphasia. Analysis was made of errors made in a standardised naming task [26]. In 4 patients no positive evidence was elicited of impairment on either a semantic or phonological level. These patients did not produce 'wrong' words, but simply failed to respond, consistent with their reduced speech output. In 1 patient only, literal paraphasic errors occurred in naming, similar to those seen in the non-fluent aphasic group. Indeed, in that patient spontaneous speech was also disordered. Speech was non-fluent with a stuttering quality, agrammatic and contained phonemic paraphasias. In 14 patients (74%), naming tasks elicited generic responses and semantic category errors, similar to those seen in the fluent aphasic group.

Thus, in terms of frequency of occurrence of linguistic features, DFT would seem to have more in common with the fluent, semantic disorder of progressive aphasia. There are however problems in interpreting the significance of verbal/semantic errors in DFT patients. A verbal response 'dog' for 'horse' may indeed reflect an underlying semantic disorder and suggest that the patient no longer has a conceptual distinction between the two animals. Alternatively, it may underscore the patient's cursory mode of responding, with lack of effort or concern for precision of responses. The presence of 'semantic errors' may therefore give rise to an overestimate in this population of the frequency of semantic disorder. Nevertheless, evidence across a range of tasks suggests that at least in a proportion of patients semantic disorder does indeed emerge with disease progression.

In a task which required patients to classify animals, 2 patients made frequent errors in naming dogs as cats and vice versa. Yet they generated both words spontaneously, so that responses cannot readily be construed as artifacts of minimal effort responding. In matching a spoken word with a picture from an array of pictures, those patients were consistent in making within but not between category matching errors (e.g. the word 'carrot' was matched with a picture of mushrooms but not a donkey). Errors secondary to apathy and lack of mental effort might be expected to elicit a rather more random distribution of errors. One patient provided explicit evidence of semantic disorder in defining words. For example, when asked to describe a carrot, she replied 'You eat it. It's sweet and covered in chocolate'. The elaborated response again suggests a genuine loss of meaning rather than lack of mental effort in responding. The patient's family had observed that she no longer appeared to understand the meaning of common words nor recognized the significance of objects.

Language Features of DFT in Progressive Aphasia

Patients with progressive aphasia, regardless of language profile, appear to share with DFT a gradual reduction in speech output leading to mutism. One patient only, who is still in the relatively early phase of disease and has a semantic disorder associated with fluent speech

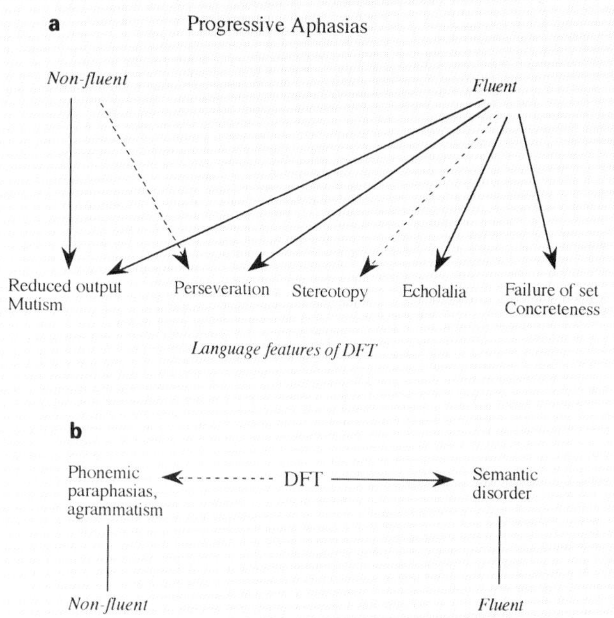

Fig. 1. Diagrams showing (**a**) features found in patients with the non-fluent and fuent forms of progressive aphasia which are characteristic of DFT, and (**b**) features found in DFT patients which are characteristic of the non-fluent and fluent forms of progressive aphasia. Solid lines indicate a strong relationship (frequent finding), whereas dotted lines indicate a weak relationship (infrequent finding).

output, currently exhibits a press of speech, which is unmonitored and stereotyped in content. Some increase in speech output has also been noted in some patients in the early stages of DFT [15]. Of the 19 patients mutism has ensued in all but 4 relatively moderately affected patients. In the non-fluent aphasic group no examples of sterotypic speech were recorded, and patients did not become echolalic. Perseverative verbal responses occurred in 2 of the 6 patients. In contrast, in the fluent group echolalia developed in 5 of the 7 patients and verbal perseverations in the entire group. Verbal stereotypies have been noted in 2 patients. In the mixed group stereotypies and perseverations were recorded in 2 patients, but there was no instances of echolalia. In the mixed group, severe comprehension impairment in some patients was not totally explicable in lexical-semantic terms and seemed to reflect failure of mental set and concreteness of thought. For example, 1 patient who failed to understand simple arithmetical questions, had no difficulty doing so provided these were couched in sentences relating to his personal work experience (i.e. sentences of greater grammatical and lexical complexity). A patient, with a fluent logorrheic speech, resembling a Wernicke type aphasia, invariably interpreted questions in mathematical terms, conforming to his former professional involvement with mathematics. (Similarly, when asked to copy line drawings, he invariably labelled the angles of all bisecting lines). That non-lexical-semantic factors were at work perhaps accounts for the surprisingly good naming performance in this and one other patient. Conceptual set failure appeared increasingly to play a role in the fluent group also, although given the breakdown in individual word semantics this could not easily be measured. The commonalities between the language disorder in the non-fluent and fluent forms of progressive aphasia and in DFT are illustrated in figure 1.

Discussion

Reports of progressive aphasia, associated with focal cerebral atrophy [1–14], highlight the diversity in the nature of the language disorder. In our own series, we have identified two prototypical profiles. In the one there is a phonological disorder, leading to impaired speech production with frequent phonemic errors. The semantic system remains relatively preserved, at least initially. In the other there is a profound impairment of the semantic system, so that the patient no longer understands word meaning (and also progressively object meaning). These two profiles are not absolute: patients vary to the extent to which they conform to the prototype. Moreover, some patients (mixed group) share features of the two, with combinations of phonological, grammatical and semantic disturbances. This third, or intermediate, group provides grounds for the assumption that the non-fluent and fluent profiles form part of a spectrum of language disorder associated with a common underlying pathology, and do not constitute discrete disease entities. The mixed group is important too in highlighting links with DFT. There was a strong suggestion in some patients that comprehension failure was influenced by 'frontal lobe' features of concreteness of thought and failure to establish mental set. Links with DFT were noted also prominently in the fluent group: echolalia and verbal perseverations occurred with comparable frequency to that in DFT.

In DFT, structural aspects of language are not the presenting nor overriding characteristic. However, there is compelling evidence that at least in a proportion of patients semantic disorder occurs, and indeed, as in patients with the fluent pattern of progressive aphasia, this may involve understanding of visual as well as verbal material. The association between DFT and fluent (semantic) aphasia is consistent with the view that both represent a fronto-temporal atrophic process: in the former the frontal lobes are the major site of pathology, with presumed increased temporal involvement with disease progression; in the latter the temporal lobes are predominantly involved, presumably with gradual spread anteriorly. What then of the association with non-fluent aphasia, in which widespread and asymmetric involvement of the left hemisphere occurs? Could this represent a separate entity as suggested by some authors [2]? It has been argued above that language profiles are not wholly discrete nor absolute, and there is overlap in symptomatology across patients, suggesting a nosological link between the different patterns. Moreover, attention should be drawn to the DFT patient, noted above, who developed a non-fluent aphasia, with stuttering output and frequent phonemic paraphasias. His pattern of language breakdown was indistinguishable from the non-fluent form of progressive aphasia. Although only 1 case amongst the group of 19, he provides evidence for an association between the bilateral fronto-temporal atrophy of DFT and the asymmetric lobar atrophy of non-fluent progressive aphasia.

In conclusion, there are commonalities between the language breakdown of DFT and the spectrum of language disorders encompassed under the rubric of 'progressive aphasia'. These findings complement the observation that patients with progressive aphasia may develop behavioural disturbance and personality change with disease progression akin to that seen in DFT. The findings support the view that DFT and progressive aphasia are part of a spectrum of clinical manifestations of non-Alzheimer lobar atrophy, which share a common pathological substrate.

References

1 Wechsler AF: Presenile dementia presenting as aphasia. J Neurol Neurosurg Psychiatry 1977; 40:303–305.
2 Mesulam MM: Slowly progressive aphasia without generalized dementia. Ann Neurol 1982;11:592–598.
3 Heath PD, Kennedy P, Kapur N: Slowly progressive aphasia without generalized dementia. Ann Neurol 1983;13:687–688.
4 Holland AL, McBurney DH, Moossy J, Reinmuth OM: The dissolution of language in Pick's disease with neurofibrillary tangles: A case study. Brain Lang 1985;24:36–58.
5 Chawluk JB, Mesulam MM, Hurtig H, et al: Slowly progressive aphasia without generalized dementia: studies with positron emission tomography. Ann Neurol 1986;19:68–74.
6 Kirshner HS, Tanridag O, Thurman L, Whetsell WO: Progressive aphasia without dementia: Two cases with focal spongiform degeneration. Ann Neurol 1987;22:527–532.
7 Poeck K, Luzzatti C: Slowly progressive aphasia in three patients: The problem of accompanying neuropsychological deficit. Brain 1988; 111:151–168.
8 Goulding PJ, Northen B, Snowden JS, et al: Progressive aphasia with right-sided extrapyramidal signs: Another manifestation of localized cerebral atrophy. J Neurol Neurosurg Psychiatry 1989;52:128–130.
9 Kempler D, Metter EJ, Riege WH, et al: Slowly progressive aphasia: Three cases with language, memory, CT and PET data. J Neurol Neurosurg Psychiatry 1990;53:987–993.
10 Delecluse F, Andersen AR, Waldemar G, et al: Cerebral blood flow in progressive aphasia without dementia. Brain 1990;113:1395–1404.
11 Tyrrell PJ, Warrington EK, Frackowiak RSJ, Rossor MN: Heterogeneity in progressive aphasia due to focal cortical atrophy. A clinical and PET study. Brain 1990;113:1321–1336.
12 Yamamoto H, Tanabe H, Kashiwagi A, et al: A case of slowly progressive aphasia without generalized dementia in a Japanese patient. Acta Neurol Scand 1990;82:102–105.
13 Kartsounis LD, Crellin RF, Crewes H, Toone BK: Primary progressive non-fluent aphasia: A case study. Cortex 1991;27:121–129.
14 Snowden JS, Neary D, Mann DMA, et al: Progressive language disorder due to lobar atrophy. Ann Neurol 1992;31:174–183.
15 Gustafson L: Frontal lobe degeneration of non-Alzheimer type. 11 Clinical picture and differential diagnosis. Arch Gerontol Geriatr 1987;6: 209–223.
16 Neary D, Snowden JS, Northen B, Goulding PJ: Dementia of frontal lobe type. J Neurol, Neurosurg Psychiatry 1988;51:353–361.
17 Mann DMA, South PW, Snowden JS, Neary D: Dementia of frontal lobe type; neuropathology and immunohistochemistry. J Neurol Neurosurg Psychiatry, in press.
18 Neary D, Snowden JS, Mann DMA, et al: Frontal lobe dementia and motor neuron disease. J Neurol Neurosurg Psychiatry 1990;53: 23–32.
19 Warrington EK, Shallice T: Category specific semantic impairments. Brain 1984;107:829–854.
20 McCarthy RA, Warrington EK: Evidence for modality specific meaning systems in the brain. Nature 1988;334:428–430.
21 Basso A, Capitani E, Laiacona M: Progressive language impairment without dementia: A case with isolated category specific semantic defect. J Neurol Neurosurg Psychiatry 1988;51:1201–1207.
22 Silveri MC, Gainotti G: Interaction between vision and language in category-specific semantic impairment. Cogn Neuropsychol 1988; 5:677–709.
23 Sartori G, Job R: The oyster with four legs: A neuropsychological study on the interaction of visual and semantic information. Cogn Neuropsychol 1988;5:105–132.
24 McKenna P, Warrington EK: Category-specific naming preservation: A single case study. J Neurol Neurosurg Psychiatry 1978;41:571–574.
25 Snowden JS, Goulding PJ, Neary D: Semantic dementia: A form of circumscribed cerebral atrophy. Behav Neurol 1989;2:167–182.
26 Kaplan E, Goodglass H, Weintraub S: The Boston Naming Test. Philadelphia, Lea & Febiger, 1983.

Dementia 1993;4:232–236

Kyle Brauer Boone
Bruce L. Miller
Ira M. Lesser

Department of Psychiatry, Harbor-UCLA Medical Center, Torrance, Calif., USA

Frontal Lobe Cognitive Functions in Aging: Methodologic Considerations

Key Words
Frontal lobe
Performance, neuropsychological
White matter lesions
Wisconsin card sorting test

Abstract
The empirical literature has been contradictory regarding whether frontal functions decline with age, perhaps due to important differences across studies in medical and psychiatric exclusion criteria. We review literature and present preliminary data suggesting that frontal lobe functions are particularly affected by several medical and psychiatric disorders common in old age. Investigations of frontal lobe functions in aging require careful screening of subject samples; otherwise, any impact of age on cognition is contaminated by the effects of coexistent physical and/or psychiatric illness.

Introduction

Within the past decade, an emerging literature has described a clinical-pathologic syndrome variously identified as dementia of the frontal lobe type [1], frontal lobe dementia of non-Alzheimer type [2], or frontal lobe degeneration [3]. Neuropsychological characteristics of this disorder primarily reflect impairment in executive or frontal lobe functions, with evolution to a diffuse dementia later in the course of the illness [1, 3]. Parallel to this literature has been the appearance of several reports suggesting that declines in frontal lobe functions are the first and most prominent cognitive impairment associated with normal aging [4–8]. Neuropsychological assessment of frontal lobe degeneration becomes problematic if the cognitive deficits associated with the disorder mimic those observed in the normal elderly population. However, we believe the case for frontal lobe decline with normal aging has been overstated due to methodological factors which will be discussed below.

Literature on Frontal Lobe Decline in Normal Aging

Declines with age in abilities subserved by the frontal lobes have received little research attention compared to examination of other abilities, such as memory, attention, processing speed, and visual spatial skills. Unfortunately, the literature which is available on frontal lobe functions in aging has been contradictory and difficult to interpret.

On the Wisconsin Card Sorting Test, reports have been divided as to whether perseverative behavior increases on this task with age; several investigators have documented significant increases in perseverative indices with age [5, 9, 10], while we [11] and others [12, 13] have failed to replicate this observation. Declines in categories completed and increases in total errors with age have been consistently reported across studies, although disagreements have emerged regarding at what age the deterioration in performance occurs. Heaton [9], Nelson [13], and Daigneault et al. [5] observed significant changes in these parameters before age 65, while we [11] did not document any significant deterioration until after age 70, and Haaland et al. [12] did not detect declines until after age 80.

Some reports [5, 14] have documented a decline in word fluency skills prior to age 80, however, other studies have presented data indicating that word generation does not decline until age 80 and later. Mittenberg et al. [6] and we [11] failed to detect significant fluency declines in subjects younger than 80, while Benton et al. [15] found a decline in word generation only after age 80, and Whelihan and Lesher [8] reported fluency declines in subjects aged 76–92 relative to 60- to 70-year-olds.

The relationship between Auditory Consonant Trigrams performance and age has been addressed in only

Kyle Brauer Boone, PhD
Department of Psychiatry
Harbor-UCLA Medical Center
1000 W. Carson Street, D-5 Annex
Torrance, CA 90509 (USA)

1013–7424/93/0044–0232
$2.75/0

one report; we [11] failed to detect any significant decreases in performance in 50- to 79-year-olds.

Whelihan and Lesher [8] and Daigneault et al. [5] noted declines with age on the Stroop interference task, although it could be argued that the poor scores could have been caused by slowing in information processing speed known to occur in the elderly. We found only a trend toward significant group differences on the interference section, but documented significant differences on word reading (Part A) and color naming (Part B) [11]. Parts A and B involve processing speed but do not require frontal abilities per se, while part C requires processing speed in conjunction with frontal inhibitory skills; thus, any declines with age on part C may simply be an artifact of declines in information processing speed. Several reports have documented declines with age on the Category test [16–20], although this finding has recently been challenged [21].

Declines with age also have been observed on some additional tests purported to be sensitive to frontal lobe integrity. Specifically, decreases with age have been reported for Porteus Mazes [5], design fluency [5, 6, 22] Hooper [8], visual reproduction subtest of the Wechsler Memory Scale [7], Self-Ordered Pointing Test [5], Visual-Verbal Test [23], and word and picture recency [6]. However, these tasks involve visual perception/spatial skills and/or memory, abilities which themselves have been documented to deteriorate with age. Thus, any declines on these tests may simply be a function of declines in these collateral, nonfrontal skills.

In summary, no definitive conclusions can be drawn from the literature on the impact of advanced age on frontal lobe functions. The reported declines on frontal lobe measures may be an artifact of deterioration in non-frontal skills needed for successful performance on the tasks. In addition, the contradictory findings across investigations may reflect important differences in medical and psychiatric status across the samples studied. The investigations varied considerably in medical and psychiatric exclusion criteria, with some reporting no exclusion criteria [7, 8, 12–14, 17], and others failing to exclude for alcoholism [7, 8, 10, 12–17, 19–22], psychiatric disturbance [7, 8, 12–14, 17, 20, 21] or medical illness [5, 7, 8, 10, 12–17, 19, 22]. Further complicating the issue, even if an attempt was made to employ appropriate exclusion criteria, subjects may have illnesses of which they are unaware. For example, although our normal elderly sample [11] was screened by interview for psychotic or major affective disorder, substance abuse, neurologic illness and significant medical illness, 18% were subsequently excluded due to positive findings on neurologic exam, significant metabolic abnormalities, and abnormal findings on EEG or MRI. Of this 18 percent, half were aged 70 or older. Exclusion criteria are of particular importance when studying frontal lobe functions given that, as will be discussed below, frontal lobe abilities appear to be particularly impacted by medical and psychiatric status.

The Relationship between Frontal Lobe Test Scores and Psychiatric and Medical Illness

A rather substantial literature has documented a relationship between psychosis and frontal lobe declines [24–27], and there is emerging evidence that depression is associated with poorer performance on such frontal lobe measures as the Wisconsin Card Sporting Test [28], Stroop Test [29], Category Test [30], and Auditory Consonant Trigrams [31]. Poor performance on frontal lobe tasks in depressed patients would be consistent with recent evidence of reduced frontal lobe blood flow [32] and glucose metabolism [33, 34] in depression. The impact of depression on neuropsychological function is particularly pertinent to the study of aging and cognition given the high rate of affective disorders in the elderly; Blazer and Williams [35] reported a prevalence rate of 14.7% for substantial depression symptoms in their community-based elderly sample.

The presence of medical illness is also known to be associated with lowered performance on cognitive tests [36], and evidence suggests that frontal lobe abilities may be particularly affected by chronic systemic illness. Willis et al. [20] found no age-related changes in performance on the Category Test in their sample of 154 healthy well-educated individuals aged 65–79 rated for the presence of chronic systemic disease. They did, however, find an association between health status and test scores, and concluded that the 'changes in executive or frontal lobe skills may be more a reflection of the increasing prevalence of illness in the elderly than a reflection of age-related brain changes' [p. 27]. Conversely, the investigators documented a significant relationship between age and memory test scores, and of interest, memory test scores were not predicted by health status.

Specific systemic illnesses which appear to be related to declines in frontal lobe abilities include hypertension, diabetes, and chronic obstructive pulmonary disease. Hypertensive patients have shown declines primarily on frontal (e.g., Category Test, Trailmaking part B), attentional, and memory tests [37, 38]. Similarly, diabetic patients have been reported to perform particularly poorly on tests requiring frontal lobe abilities of complex problem-solving and abstract reasoning [39], and to score significantly poorer on Trailmaking part B, and the Category Test [40]. Chronic obstructive pulmonary disease has been reported to be associated with decrements in perceptual-motor learning, problem solving, and motor speed and strength in the context of intact verbal intellectual abilities, alertness, and psychomotor speed [41].

The physiological mechanism underlying the sensitivity of frontal lobe functions to systemic illness has not yet been elucidated, although in some cases it may be related to decreased cerebral blood flow in anterior brain regions. For example, Waldstein et al. [38] note that the relative impairment in frontal lobe skills in hypertension is consistent with reported declines in rCBF in frontal and temporal regions in hypertensive patients. The importance of illness factors such as hypertension in the study of frontal lobe functions in the elderly becomes apparent when the prevalence of hypertension is considered. In subjects aged 65 and older, hypertension prevalence rates of between 18 and 56% have been documented for men, and between 30 and 70% for women [42].

Diseases such as hypertension and diabetes may lead to 'silent' cerebrovascular lesions in brain white matter [43–45], which also cause deficits in frontal lobe abilities. We have reported [46] that healthy elderly with total area of MRI-detected white matter lesions >10 cm^2 scored significantly below subjects with white matter lesion area <10 cm^2 on selected frontal lobe measures (Wisconsin Card Sort Test, categories and number of perseverative responses; Auditory Consonant Trigrams) and basic attention (Digit Span), even after covarying for the effects of age. In contrast, no significant declines in IQ, memory, language, visual-spatial skills, or information processing speed were associated with white matter lesions. We hypothesized, based on the work of Mesulam [47], that even though the lesions did not necessarily cluster in frontal areas, they may have produced a frontal lobe syndrome through sabotaging the integration by the frontal lobes of networks for complex behavior.

As with hypertension, the prevalence of white matter lesions in elderly is substantial. Bradley et al. [48] reported that 30% of all patients over the age of 60 had white matter lesions on MRI scanning, while in our sample of normal elderly, approximately 75% of subjects over age 70 had detectable lesions in white matter [46]. Six percent of our healthy sample had white matter lesion area of sufficient size (>10 cm^2) to be associated with significant declines in frontal and attentional tasks. We suspect that the prevalence of large areas of white matter lesions is probably much greater in the general elderly population as compared to our sample which met extensive medical exclusion criteria.

Comparison of Performance on Frontal Lobe Tests in Patients with Frontal Lobe Degeneration and in Subjects with Large Area of White Matter Lesions

To illustrate the magnitude of the decline in frontal lobe functions which can be associated with medical illness factors in 'normal' elderly, we have recently reexamined our neuropsychological data on healthy elderly with large total area of white matter lesions [47] in the context of our findings on patients with frontal lobe degeneration. As we have previously published, our neuropsychological evaluation of 6 patients with frontal dobe degeneration (FLD) revealed selective impairment relative to 6 education- and age-matched controls in frontal lobe abilities, attentional skills, and overall intellectual level, with relative sparing of language, memory and visual-spatial skills [3]. Similarly, as discussed above, our comparison of 6 healthy elderly with white matter lesions (WML) area >10 cm^2 versus subjects with WML area <10 cm^2 revealed declines in selected frontal lobe tasks and attention in the context of normal intelligence, visual spatial skills, memory, and information processing speed. We were struck by the similar profile of neuropsychological deficits in the FLD and WML groups, and have subsequently computed Kruskal-Wallis analyses comparing the 6 FLD patients with their 6 controls and the 6 subjects with WML area >10 cm^2.

As shown in table 1, significant group differences were observed for several neuropsychological scores, including IQ, frontal lobe tasks (Auditory Consonant Trigrams, Verbal Fluency, perseverative responses on the Wisconsin Card Sorting Test) and attention (Digit Span). Post-hoc comparisons indicated that the significant group differences were due to discrepancies in performance between the controls and the two other groups. No significant differences were observed between the FLD and WML groups, although the small sample sizes may have limited the power of the analyses to detect significant group differences. Inspection of the group means suggested that the WML group obtained higher mean scores than the FLD patients on most test scores, however, of interest, on three frontal and attentional measures (Auditory Consonant Trigrams, perseverative responses on the Wisconsin Card Sorting Test, Digit Span), the means for the FLD and WML groups were almost identical. These data might suggest that while older subjects with WML may not be as impaired on IQ, memory, or visual spatial performance as FLD patients, on selected frontal lobe and attentional tasks the two groups appear virtually indistinguishable.

While the idea that patients with FLD and normal elderly with large area of WML may show a similar magnitude of impairment on frontal lobe and attentional tasks is intriguing, these findings need to be viewed as tentative given the small sample sizes, multiple comparisons, and inability to covary for age and educational differences due to the limitations of nonparametric analyses. In addition, it is important to note that the FLD and WML subjects were not studied with identical imaging techniques, so it remains unclear to what extent these two groups may overlap in terms of structural and functional brain abnormalities. However, the data which are available would suggest that the two groups are distinct. For example, formal quantification of WML areas was not available on the six FLD patients, although visual inspection of MRI scans of these patients showed only 1 subject with large area of WML. Similarly, only 2 of the 6 elderly with large area of WML had SPECT exams, but both of these studies revealed normal blood flow in contrast to the consistent evidence of bilateral frontal lobe hypoperfusion in the FLD patients.

Table 1. Neuropsychological performance in patients with FLD, subjects with large area of WML, and controls

	FLD (n = 6)	WML > 10 cm² (n = 6)	Controls (n = 6)	p[1]
Age	63.0 ± 8.3	71.7 ± 4.9	62.7 ± 7.6	0.050
Education	17.5 ± 2.2	13.3 ± 1.5	14.8 ± 2.9	0.019[a]
FSIQ	92.0 ± 18.6	106.7 ± 8.7	125.2 ± 7.5	0.003[b]
Frontal				
WCST Categories	1.7 ± 2.4	2.8 ± 2.3	4.7 ± 2.2	0.091
WCST Pers. Resp.	55.0 ± 36.7	57.5 ± 45.8	16.5 ± 18.6	0.031[b]
ACT	29.6 ± 13.4	33.8 ± 10.7	50.5 ± 8.8	0.018[b]
Stroop 3	207.8 ± 86.6	171.0 ± 69.7	133.0 ± 73.9	0.204
FAS	18.7 ± 16.5	30.7 ± 8.3	51.3 ± 19.0	0.018[c]
Attention				
Digit Span	8.3 ± 2.7	8.7 ± 1.9	12.8 ± 1.5	0.014[b]
Visuospatial				
R-O copy	29.2 ± 4.9	33.5 ± 0.8	33.0 ± 2.4	0.085
Memory				
WMS LM % ret.	52.8 ± 42.5	74.2 ± 18.5	85.2 ± 9.3	0.207
WMS VR % ret.	34.6 ± 40.9	58.8 ± 27.4	64.5 ± 30.2	0.383

WCST= Wisconsin Card Sorting Test.
1 Kruskal-Wallis analyses.
a FLD versus WML; b control versus FLD and WML; c control versus FLD.

Conclusion

We strongly suspect that the purported declines in frontal lobe functioning with age, and particularly the reported increases in perseverative behavior with advanced age, are to a substantial degree related to the presence of psychiatric disorder (e.g., depression), systemic illness and/or white matter lesions in the older samples studied.

Clearly, our findings indicate that any investigation of frontal lobe functions in aging requires careful screening of subject samples; otherwise, any impact of age on cognition is contaminated by the effects of coexistent physical and/or psychiatric illness. Of concern, even when exclusion criteria are used, a substantial percent of subjects may have medical conditions of which they are unaware. Thus, not only should older subjects be carefully questioned for history of medical illness, but comprehensive imaging, physical examination, and laboratory studies are needed to insure the health of the sample studied.

Acknowledgments

This work was supported in part by a State of California, Department of Mental Health Contract (90-70042) (to I.M.L), by a grant from the National Institute of Mental Health (MH43960) (to I.M.L), and by a grant from the National Institute of Aging (UCLA Alzheimer Disease Center, AG10123) (to B.L.M.).

References

1 Neary D, Snowden JS, Northen B, Goulding P: Dementia of frontal lobe type. J Neurol Neurosurg Psychiatry 1988;51:353–361.

2 Gustafson L, Brun A, Risberg J: Frontal lobe dementia of non-Alzheimer type; in Wurtman RJ, Corkin S, Growdon J, Ritter-Walker E (eds): Alzheimer's Disease. Advances in Neurology. New York, Raven Press, 1990, vol 51, pp 65–71.

3 Miller BL, Cummings JL, Villanueva-Meyer J, Boone K, Mehringer CM, Lesser IM, Mena I: Frontal lobe degeneration: Clinical, neuropsychological, and SPECT characteristics. Neurology 1991;41:1374–1382.

4 Albert MS, Kaplan E: Organic implications of neuropsychological deficits in the elderly; in Poon LW, Fozard JL, Cermak LS, Arenberg D, Thompson LW (eds): New Directions in Memory and Aging: Proceedings of the George A. Talland Memorial Conference. Hillsdale, Erlbaum, 1980.
5 Daigneault S, Braun CMJ, Whitaker HA: Early effects of normal aging in perseverative and non-perseverative prefrontal measures. Dev Neuropsychol 1992;8:99–114.
6 Mittenberg W, Seidenberg M, O'Leary DS, DiGiulio DV: Changes in cerebral functioning associated with normal aging. J Clin Exp Neuropsychol 1989;11:918–932.
7 Veroff AE: The neuropsychology of aging: Qualitative analysis of visual reproductions. Psychol Res 1980;41:259–268.
8 Whelihan WM, Lesher EL: Neuropsychological changes in frontal functions with aging. Dev Neuropsychol 1985;1:371–380.
9 Heaton RK: Wisconsin Card Sorting Test Manual. Odessa, Psychological Assessment Resources, 1981.
10 Loranger AW, Misiak H: The performance of aged females on five non-language tests of intellectual functions. J Clin Psychol 1960;16: 189–191.
11 Boone KB, Miller BL, Lesser IM, Hill E, D'Elia L: Performance on frontal lobe tests in healthy, older individuals. Dev Neuropsychol 1990;6: 215–223.
12 Haaland KY, Vranes LF, Goodwin JS, Garry PJ: Wisconsin Card Sort Test performance in a healthy elderly population. J Gerontol 1987; 42:345–346.
13 Nelson HE: A modified card sorting test sensitive to frontal lobe defects. Cortex 1976;12: 313–324.
14 Furry CA, Baltes PB: The effect of age differences in ability-extraneous performance variables on the assessment of intelligence in children, adults, and the elderly. J Gerontol 1973; 28:73–80.
15 Benton AL, Eslinger PJ, Damasio AR: Normative observations on neuropsychological test performances in old age. J Clin Neuropsychol 1981;3:33–42.
16 Fromm-Auch D, Yeudall LT: Normative data for the Halstead-Reitan Neurological Tests. J Clin Neuropsychol 1983;5:221–238.
17 Macks JL, Carlson NJ: Conceptual deficits and aging: The Category Test. Percept Mot Skills 1978;46:123–128.
18 Pauker JD: 'Norms' (or standards) for the Halstead-Reitan Neuropsychological Test battery, based on a nonclinical, adult sample. Paper presented at the Annual Convention of the Canadian Psychological Association, Calgary, 1980.
19 Reed HBC, Reitan RM: A comparison of the effects of the normal aging process with the effects of organic brain-damage on adaptive abilities. J Gerontol 1963;18:177–179.
20 Wood WG, Elias MF, Schultz NR, Pentz CA: Age differences in neuropsychological performance among healthy well-educated subjects. J Clin Exp Gerontol 1980;2:141–158.
21 Willis L, Yeo RA, Thomas P, Garry PJ: Differential declines in cognitive function with aging: The possible role of health status. Dev Neuropsychol 1988;4:23–28.
22 Ruff RM, Light RH, Evans RW: The Ruff Figural Fluency Test: A normative study with adults. Dev Neuropsychol 1987;3:37–51.
23 Albert MS, Wolfe J, Lafleche G: Differences in abstraction ability with age. Psychol Aging 1990;5:94–100.
24 Lesser IM, Miller BL, Boone KB, Hill-Gutierrez E, Mehringer CM, Wong K, Mena I: Brain injury and cognitive function in late-onset psychotic depression. J Neuropsychiatr Clin Neurosci 1991;3:33–40.
25 Miller BL, Lesser IM, Boone KB, Hill E, Mehringer CM, Wong K: Brain lesions and cognitive function in late-life psychosis. Br J Psychiatry 1991;158:76–82.
26 Weinberger DR, Berman KF, Daniel DG: Prefrontal cortex dysfunction in schizophrenia; in Levin HS, Eisenberg HM, Benton AL (eds): Frontal Lobe Function and Dysfunction. New York, Oxford University Press, 1991 pp 275–287.
27 Weinberger DR, Berman KF, Zec RF: Physiologic dysfunction of dorsolateral prefrontal cortex in schizophrenia. I. Regional cerebral blood flow evidence (rCBF). Arch Gen Psychiatry 1986;43:114–125.
28 Martin DJ, Oren Z, Boone K: Major depressives' and dysthymics' performance on the Wisconsin Card Sorting Test. J Clin Psychol 1991;47:684–690.
29 Raskin A, Friedman AS, DiMascio A: Cognitive and performance deficits in depression. Psychopharmacology Bull 18:196–202.
30 Savard RJ, Rey AC, Post RM: Halstead-Reitan Category Test in bipolar and unipolar affective disorders: Relationship to age and phase in illness. J Nerv Ment Dis 1980;168:297–304.
31 Cohen RM, Weingartner H, Smallberg SA, Pickar D, Murphy DL: Effort and cognition in depression. Arch Gen Psychiatry 1982;39:593–597.
32 Mayberg HS, Jeffery PJ, Wagner HN, Simpson SG: Regional cerebral blood flow in patients with refractory unipolar depression measured with TC-99m HMPAO SPECT. J Nucl Med 1991;32:951.
33 Hurwitz TA, Clark C, Murphy E, Klonoff H, Martin WRW, Pate BD: Regional cerebral glucose metabolism in major depressive disorder. Can J Psychiatry 1990;35:684–688.
34 Baxter LR, Schwartz JM, Phelps ME, Mazziotta JC, Guze BH, Selin CE, Gerner RH, Sumida RM: Reduction of prefrontal cortex glucose metabolism common to three types of depression. Arch Gen Psychiatry 1989;46:243–250.
35 Blazer D, Williams CD: Epidemiology of dysphoria and depression in an elderly population. Am J Psychiatry 1980;137:439–444.
36 Tarter RE, Edwards KL, Van Thiel DH: Perspective and rationale for neuropsychological assessment of medical disease; in Tarter RE, Van Thiel DH, Edwards KL (eds): Medical Neuropsychology: The Impact of Disease on Behavior. New York, Plenum Press, 1988, pp 1–10.
37 Elias MF, Robbins MA, Schultz NR, Streeten DHP: A longitudinal study of neuropsychological test performance of hypertensive and normotensive adults: Initial findings. J Gerontol 1986;41:503–505.
38 Waldstein SR, Manuck SB, Ryan CM, Muldoon MF: Neuropsychological correlates fo hypertension: Review and methodologic considerations. Psychol Bull 1991;110:451–468.
39 Rennick PM, Wilder RM, Sargent J, Ashley BJ: Retinopathy as an indicator of cognitive-perceptual-motor impairment in diabetic adults (summary). Proc 76th Annu Convent Am Psychol Assoc 1968, vol 3, pp 473–474.
40 Skenazy JA, Bigler ED: Neuropsychological findings in diabetes mellitus. J Clin Psychol 1984;40:246–258.
41 Prigatano GP, Levin DC: Pulmonary system; in Tarter RE, Van Thiel DH, Edwards KL (eds): Medical Neuropsychology: The Impact of Disease on Behavior. New York, Plenum Press, 1988, pp 11–26.
42 Bots ML, Grobbee DE, Hofman A: High blood pressure in the elderly. Epidemiol Rev 1991; 13:294–314.
43 Schmidt R, Fazekas F, Kleinert G, Offenbacher H, Gindl K, Payer F, Freidl W, Niederkorn K, Lechner H: Magnetic resonance imaging signal hyperintensities in the deep and subcortical white matter. Arch Neurol 1992;49: 825–827.
44 Awad IA, Spoetzler RF, Hodak JA, Awad CA, Carey RC: Incidental subcortical lesions identified on magnetic resonance imaging in the elderly. I. Correlation with age and cerebrovascular risk factors. Stroke 1986;17:1084–1089.
45 Roman GC: Senile dementia of the Binswanger type: A vascular form of dementia in the elderly. JAMA 1987;258:1782–1788.
46 Boone KB, Miller BL, Lesser IM, Mehringer CM, Hill-Gutierrez EH, Goldberg MA, Berman NG: Neuropsychological correlates of white-matter lesions in healthy elderly subjects: A threshold effect. Arch Neurol 1992;49:549–554.
47 Mesulam M: Large-scale neurocognitive networks and distributed processing for attention, language, and memory. Ann Neurol 1990;28: 597–613.
48 Bradley WG, Waluch V, Brant-Zawadszki M: Patchy periventricular white matter lesions in the elderly: A common observation during NMR imaging. Noninvasive Med Imaging 1984;1:35–41.